D1591632

Adaptation to Changing Health

Adaptation to Changing Health

Response Shift in Quality-of-Life Research

Edited by
Carolyn E. Schwartz
Mirjam A. G. Sprangers

American Psychological Association
Washington, DC

Published by
American Psychological Association
750 First Street, NE
Washington, DC 20002

Copies may be ordered from
APA Order Department
P.O. Box 92984
Washington, DC 20090-2984

In the U.K., Europe, Africa, and the Middle East, copies may be ordered from
American Psychological Association
3 Henrietta Street
Covent Garden, London
WC2E 8LU England

Typeset in Century Schoolbook by EPS Group Inc., Easton, MD

Printer: Automated Graphics Systems, White Plains, MD
Cover Designer: Naylor design, Washington, DC
Technical/Production Editor: Jennifer Powers

Library of Congress Cataloging-in-Publication Data
Adaptation to changing health : response shift in quality-of-life research / edited by Carolyn E. Schwartz and Mirjam A. G. Sprangers.
p. ; cm.
Includes bibliographical references and indexes.
ISBN 1-55798-710-6 (case : alk. paper)
1. Sick—Psychology. 2. Quality of life. 3. Health behavior.
4. Medicine and psychology. I. Schwartz, Carolyn E.
II. Sprangers, Mirjam A. G.
[DNLM: 1. Adaptation, Psychological. 2. Attitude to Health. 3. Life Change Events. 4. Quality of Life. 5. Research. BF 335 A2205 2000]
R726.5.A334 2000
155.9′3—dc21

00-025296

British Library Cataloguing-in-Publication Data
A CIP record is available from the British Library.

Printed in the United States of America
First Edition

To David and Abraham Waldman and Theo Jonkergouw,
who enhance the quality of our lives

Contents

Contributors

Jenny Broersen, MA, Psychiatric Centre Joris, Delft, the Netherlands

John P. Browne, PhD, Department of Psychology, Royal College of Surgeons in Ireland, Dublin, Ireland

Lawren H. Daltroy, DrPH, RBB Multipurpose Arthritis and Musculoskeletal Diseases Center, Brigham and Women's Hospital; Department of Rheumatology, Immunology, and Allergy, Brigham and Women's Hospital; Harvard Medical School, Department of Medicine, Department of Health and Social Behavior, Harvard School of Public Health, Boston, MA, USA

Frits S. A. M. van Dam, PhD, Division of Psychosocial Research and Epidemiology, Netherlands Cancer Institute, Amsterdam, the Netherlands

Holley M. Eaton, BSN, MA, RBB Multipurpose Arthritis and Musculoskeletal Diseases Center, Brigham and Women's Hospital, Boston, MA, USA

David T. Eton, PhD, Department of Psychology, Carnegie Mellon University, Pittsburgh, PA, USA

Susan Folkman, PhD, University of California at San Francisco, Center for AIDS Prevention Studies, San Francisco, CA, USA

Leslie A. Lenert, MD, MS, Section on Health Services Research, Department of Veterans Affairs Health Care System; Department of Medicine, University of California San Diego, San Diego, CA, USA

Stephen J. Lepore, PhD, Department of Psychology, Brooklyn College of the City of New York, Brooklyn, NY, USA

Matthew H. Liang, MD, MPH, RBB Multipurpose Arthritis and Musculoskeletal Diseases Center, Brigham and Women's Hospital; Department of Rheumatology, Immunology, and Allergy, Brigham and Women's Hospital; Harvard Medical School, Department of Medicine; Department of Health Policy and Management, Harvard School of Public Health, Boston, MA, USA

Hilary A. Llewellyn-Thomas, PhD, Clinical Epidemiology Unit, Sunnybrook & Women's College Health Science Centre; Department of Nursing Science, University of Toronto, Toronto, Ontario, Canada; and Center for the Clinical Evaluative Sciences, Department of Community and Family Medicine, Dartmouth Medical School, Dartmouth, NH, USA.

Litanja Lodder, MA, Department of Medical Psychology and Psychotherapy, Erasmus University Rotterdam, Rotterdam, the Netherlands

Hanna M. McGee, PhD, Department of Psychology, Royal College of Surgeons in Ireland, Dublin, Ireland

Ciaran A. O'Boyle, PhD, Department of Psychology, Royal College of Surgeons in Ireland, Dublin, Ireland

Paul Oosterveld, PhD, Department of Medical Psychology, the Academic Medical Center, University of Amsterdam, Amsterdam, the Netherlands

Allen Parducci, PhD, Department of Psychology (Emeritus), University of California at Los Angeles, Los Angeles, CA, USA

Charlotte B. Phillips, RN, MPH, RBB Multipurpose Arthritis and Musculoskeletal Diseases Center, Brigham and Women's Hospital, Boston, MA, USA

Bruce D. Rapkin, PhD, Department of Psychiatry and the Behavioral Sciences, Memorial Sloane-Kettering Cancer Center, New York, NY, USA

T. Anne Richards, MA, University of California at San Francisco, Center for AIDS Prevention Studies, San Francisco, CA, USA

Carolyn E. Schwartz, ScD, Frontier Science and Technology Research Foundation, Inc.; Department of Psychiatry, Beth Israel Deaconess Medical Center, Harvard Medical School, Boston, MA. Currently: Department of Family Medicine and Community Health, University of Massachusetts Medical School, Worcester, MA, USA

Meir Sendor, PhD, Young Israel of Sharon, Sharon, MA; Department of Near Eastern and Judaic Studies, Brandeis University, Waltham, MA, USA

Ellen Smets, PhD, Department of Medical Psychology, the Academic Medical Center, University of Amsterdam, Amsterdam, the Netherlands

Mirjam A. G. Sprangers, PhD, Department of Medical Psychology, the Academic Medical Center, University of Amsterdam, Amsterdam, the Netherlands

Jonathan R. Treadwell, PhD, Division of Clinical Pharmacology, Department of Medicine, Stanford University School of Medicine, Stanford, CA, USA

Mechteld R. M. Visser, PhD, Department of Medical Psychology, the Academic Medical Center, University of Amsterdam, Amsterdam, the Netherlands

Lidwina Wever, Division of Psychosocial Research and Epidemiology, Netherlands Cancer Institute, Amsterdam, the Netherlands

Ira B. Wilson, MD, MSc, Department of Clinical Care Research and the Department of Medicine, New England Medical Center, Boston, MA, USA

Acknowledgments

We would like to acknowledge the many investigators in the social and medical sciences whose interest and excitement have made pursuing response shift investigations an enjoyable challenge. We would first like to thank the social and medical scientists who participated in the Response Shift Workshop held in Boston, December 1996. These invaluable colleagues have advanced the conceptualization of response shift phenomena and stimulated our thinking about its theoretical and methodological implications. The workshop participants were as follows: Achilles A. Armenakis, PhD; Katy Benjamin, SM, MSW, DrPH; Lawren H. Daltroy, DrPH; Susan Folkman, PhD; Maureen Genderson, PhD; Rick Gibbons, PhD; Hanneke C. J. M. de Haes, PhD; Hang Lee, PhD; Geraldine V. Padilla, PhD; Allen Parducci, PhD; Bruce Rapkin, PhD; Patricia Rieker, PhD; Rabbi Meir Sendor, PhD; and Ira Wilson, MD, MSc. We would like to thank Rebecca Feinberg for her conscientious assistance with manuscript preparation.

Dr. Schwartz is also indebted to Marvin Zelen, PhD, and Thelma Zelen for their generous support; to Bruce Rapkin, PhD, for his enthusiasm and assistance in thinking through some of the intricacies and implications of response shift phenomena; and to the research study patients as well as family and friends who died of cancer, whose experience and example influenced her thinking about response shift phenomena. She would like to acknowledge the financial support from the Agency for Health Care Policy and Research (Grant RO1 HSO8582-03) and Frontier Science and Technology Research Foundation, Inc.

Dr. Sprangers would also like to express her gratitude to Frits van Dam, PhD, who saw the relevance of response shift for cancer research and health psychology. She is further indebted to Hanneke de Haes, PhD, for many inspiring discussions about response shift and her continuous support and stimulation to pursue response shift research. Finally, she would like to thank her other colleagues of the Department of Medical Psychology for their enthusiasm, critical thinking, and support.

Introduction

The field of quality-of-life (QOL) research has burgeoned in the last two decades. The prevalence of peer-reviewed journal articles and books on the topic has risen dramatically, and the inclusion of QOL measures in health-related research has become the standard. In this context, QOL refers to the physical, social, psychological, and existential aspects of well-being that might be affected by the disease and its treatment. Concomitant, albeit unrelated, to this increased acceptance, is a growth in the complexity and sophistication of psychometric methods for evaluating new measurement tools (e.g., item response theory, structural equation modeling, etc.). Despite these parallel advances, the field of QOL research is facing a watershed: There exists an awareness that QOL research often yields findings that do not make sense, are paradoxical, cannot help clinical and social sciences researchers identify the better treatment between two or more clinically equivalent options, or cannot help us understand how people perceive their QOL over time. That is to say, QOL research frequently seems to lack sensitivity to the subtleties or complexity inherent in human behavior.

The construct of response shift represents a promising avenue of development for those clinical and social sciences researchers who seek to integrate these conceptual and psychometric complexities and hence to deepen their work. Response shift is of particular importance when individuals undergo a change in health state. The working definition of *response shift* states that when individuals undergo a change in health state, they may change their internal standards, their values, or their conceptualization of QOL (the construct is fully articulated in chapters 1 and 6). These changes are also referred to as recalibration, reprioritization, and reconceptualization response shifts, respectively.[1]

Thus, the construct refers to a dynamic process that has important implications for measurement. That is to say, if an individual changes internal standards, values, or conceptualization of QOL over the course of time, then answers to the same items by the same individual may not be as comparable over time as originally thought. This is a problem that many clinicians recognize and that often leads them to nod their heads and confess that for this reason, they find QOL research less meaningful than they had hoped. In contrast to the clinicians' head nodding, many researchers shake their heads in grave concern: The emergence of response shift may threaten the validity of the assumptions and thus the foundation of their modus operandi, the self-report measure. Indeed, if response shift proves to be a viable concept, it can enhance an understand-

[1]In the interest of ensuring that each chapter of the book can be read independently, this working definition is repeated throughout the book.

ing of how patients perceive their QOL over time, as well as lead us to enhance our methods of assessing change in QOL. Thus response shift may represent a paradigm shift for self-report measurement.

This concentrated tome explores the theoretical, methodological, and empirical implications of response shift to guide further development of this construct/phenomenon in QOL research. In addition to including reprints or adaptations of previously published seminal articles on response shift, the book includes a number of new theoretical and empirical contributions. The first part of the book, "Theoretical Reflections," provides a theoretical foundation for response shift work by elucidating constructs and mechanisms that have developed thus far in social sciences research. Chapters in this part examine evidence of response shift among bereaved caregivers to people with AIDS, patients with prostate cancer, and people living with AIDS. The part begins with a chapter (1) that presents a theoretical model to explain the presence or absence of response shift as a result of a catalyst and the interaction of antecedents and mechanisms. Whereas antecedents refer to stable characteristics of the individual, mechanisms entail behavioral, cognitive, and affective processes to adjust to the catalytic health state change. The interaction of antecedents and mechanisms leads to response shifts, which are postulated to affect perceived QOL.

The other chapters in the first part address and expand the theoretical framework for response shift phenomena in various populations and regarding different antecedents and mechanisms. In chapter 2, Richards and Folkman address response shifts among bereaved caregivers from a coping perspective. Lepore and Eton (chapter 3) compare the fit of suppressor and buffering models using data that operationalize recalibration and reprioritization response shifts in patients with prostate cancer. Rapkin's chapter (4) focuses on how goal setting and changes in goals over the course of disease elicit reprioritization response shift and how this inclusion of response shift explains more variance in perceived QOL. Thus each chapter confronts some of the conceptual intricacies of the model that we have proposed. The integrative discussion (chapter 5) highlights the theoretical issues that merit elucidation.

In the second part, "Methodological Pathways," existing and new methods for assessing response shift are examined, and methodological considerations for distinguishing response shift from measurement artifact are discussed. Data using examples of individualized methods and design approaches are also presented. In chapter 6, we present a host of methods for assessing response shift, some of which involve primary data collection and others of which utilize recent quantitative methods. We also recommend a reexamination of some of the tenets of psychometric theory. A number of the suggested methods are exemplified using empirical data in the subsequent chapters. In chapter 7, Llewellyn-Thomas and Schwartz provide guidelines to distinguish response shift from systematic biases when studying patients' preferences for different health states. O'Boyle,

McGee, and Browne (chapter 8) focus on the Schedule for Evaluation of Individual Quality of Life as an example of the individualized measures, and Sprangers et al. (chapter 9) exemplify the use of the thentest as a design approach for assessing response shift. The integrative discussion (chapter 10) examines some of the conundrums facing this emerging area of investigation. Thus each chapter contributes to an understanding of the methodological pathways to assess response shift or exemplifies some of the available tools for examining response shift in QOL data.[2]

The third part of the book, "New Perspectives on Existing Data," focuses on the implications of response shift for clinical research by presenting discussions of existing paradoxes of clinical and policy research that can be elucidated by response shift. In chapter 11, Wilson provides a clinical understanding and clinical context for the concept of response shift, by discussing the relationship between response shift and intriguing issues in clinical care, such as somatization, hypochondriasis, placebo effects, and the physician–patient relationship. The subsequent chapters reveal response shift phenomena using secondary analyses of existing data. Schwartz and Sendor (chapter 12) present data on the psychosocial benefits of altruistic behavior and suggest that response shift is a mechanism by which these benefits accrue. Daltroy et al. (chapter 13) present empirical data to illustrate how a paradoxical discrepancy between objective and subjective indicators of health can be explained by response shift. Finally, in chapter 14, Lenert et al. challenge a common practice in cost-effectiveness analysis by showing that patients' life and treatment experiences interact with their preferences. The integrative discussion (chapter 15) highlights the implications and directions for future research on response shift.

When the models and methods of assessing response shift phenomena presented in this book are validated and honed, it would seem likely that we will be better able to understand and assess experienced QOL over time. Chapter 4, for example, shows how measuring reprioritization response shift increased the amount of explained variance in QOL outcomes among people with AIDS. Chapter 13 illustrates how considering recalibration response shift may improve the correlation between subjective and objective assessments of functional status. Thus these preliminary investigations support the idea that considering response shift phenomena can improve our understanding and thus our ability to predict experienced QOL over time. Future research might build on this preliminary foundation to examine the contexts in which response shift phenomena are useful or not useful for understanding QOL over time.

With this brief introduction, we invite the reader to enjoy the new path that this emerging construct opens for clinical and psychosocial investigators of health-related QOL, as well as for any researcher for whom

[2]It should be noted that, although it is not their primary focus, selected chapters in the other parts of this book also present empirical data on response shift, including chapters 2, 3, 4, 12, 13, and 14.

self-report data play a primary role. We trust that we face the beginning of a new line of research, one that offers exciting opportunities for investigation, collaboration, and contribution to the understanding of how people experience their QOL over time. By approaching this emerging construct in QOL and outcomes research from theoretical, methodological, and applied vantage points, this tome is intended to stimulate the investigation of response shift phenomena among researchers from health psychology, health services, and medical research.

Adaptation to Changing Health

An Historical Introduction to Response Shift

Allen Parducci

The concept of response shift is grounded in the history of a special kind of psychological relativism, a relativism in which the judged value of any experience depends on its current place in a changing context of related experiences. This species of relativism has a long history. We find it already in Plato, some 2,400 years ago. In Book IX of *The Republic*, Socrates asserted that people feel pain when in fact they are only shifting from a pleasurable state to a more neutral state and that they feel pleasure when shifting from a painful to a more neutral state. Plato was particularly concerned with distinguishing between experienced shifts and what he thought was the true, underlying, unchanging reality. Although identified by other terms, this distinction has loomed large in the subsequent history of response shift. It is still around today.

No one would deny that what seems like the very same condition can at one time be satisfying and at another time dissatisfying. The same little apartment that seemed so wonderful when we first established an independent household would now seem impossibly cramped and unlivable. In the other direction, the same degree of physical deterioration that would once have been depressing may now allow us to experience a renewed sense of our own animal vigor.

As in the Platonic dialogues between Socrates and the Sophists in Athens, there continues to be a disparity of interests between those who are concerned with shifts in experience and those who are concerned with the true, unchanging reality, regardless of how it is experienced. Plato sometimes treated subjective experience as trivial, a shadowy distortion of the real world of pure ideas. So, too, are economists concerned with what they call "utilities," those relatively unchanging values measured by marketplace exchanges and dollar values, rather than with the transitory elations and disappointments that are actually experienced, such as the varying degrees of personal satisfaction or pleasure. Psychologists differ with respect to these concerns, but the contributors to this volume are among those most interested in what self-reports reveal about subjective experiences. In the field of health, we are sometimes as concerned with changes in how patients feel as with the more strictly physical aspects of their medical conditions. An important objective of therapy may be to facilitate changes in the way particular states are experienced, changes not only in standards but also in values and conceptualizations. This is the thrust of response shift theory.

Scientific Roots

The history of psychology as a self-proclaimed "science" begins in the 19th century with attempts to relate perceptual experience to attributes of the physical world. The Weber and Fechner Laws are the best known examples. Both of these laws describe response shifts in which a particular physical difference between stimuli is more likely to be discriminated or to seem larger when the absolute values of the stimuli are smaller. This emphasis on stimulus relationships was lost in the heyday of classical introspection, at the end of the 19th century, when controlled laboratory experiments were designed to find simple one-to-one connections between physical stimuli and subjective experiences. In their revolt against the subjective character of introspectionism, behaviorists retained the notion of one-to-one connections; however, behaviorists substituted connections between stimulus and response (i.e., habits) for the introspectionists' connections between stimulus and subjective experience. Some of this difference in approach has been preserved in the extensive literature on scaling, which, although compatible with response shifts, tends to emphasize an underlying constancy. For example, Thurstone showed how constant scale values of stimuli could be inferred from data in which the ratings of the stimuli were changing systematically (see Torgerson, 1958). Anderson (1981) and Birnbaum (1982) have relied on constancy of scale values to test algebraic models of cognitive processes. However, the search for constancies should not obscure the real changes in what is experienced.

Another highly sophisticated precursor to response shift theory can be found in signal detection theory (see Green & Swets, 1966) which explains how systematic changes in the probability of identifying the presence of a stimulus or a disease vary with shifts in the criterion or standard: An increasing probability of hits is accompanied by an increasing probability of false alarms. This has proven enormously influential for medical decisions in that it is now universally recognized that a particular diagnostic test may identify most victims of a disease but at a price of too many false diagnoses of the presence of the disease in patients who do not have it. The various contributions to the present book have the potential of producing a related but much more widely applicable effect on the interpretation of medical data, alerting researchers to the ubiquitous influence that changing standards may have on test results.

The present concern with response shifts seems close in spirit to Gestalt psychology for which the central thesis is that our perceptual system responds to relationships between stimuli rather than to the absolute characteristics of a stimulus. Thus a response to a particular stimulus shifts with changes in surrounding stimulation (e.g., Wallach, 1948). This is generalized in the work of Helson (1964) whose theory of adaptation level asserts that the judgment of any stimulus, whether a particular visual hue or level of health, depends on how it compares with an average of other stimuli, whether recently presented hues or prior levels of health. This level of adaptation functions as a single-valued standard for judgment.

Recently experienced stimuli constitute the more general, many-valued context for judgment, with *context* defined as the set of those stimulus values, real or imaginary, that affect the judgment. Simple psychophysical experiments in which participants rate some aspect of each of a succession of presented stimuli, such as the heaviness of lifted weights, have demonstrated repeatedly the advantages of taking account of the entire set of presented stimuli rather than just their mean or adaptation level. For example, the experienced heaviness of each successive weight can be predicted more accurately when account is taken of the place of that weight in the frequency distribution of all the weights that have been presented during the experimental session. Given this context of closely related stimuli, the judgment of any stimulus within that context is precisely determined. My own range-frequency theory of judgment provides a quantitative basis for predicting shifts in judgments of stimuli with shifts in their context (Parducci, 1995).

However, it is clear that outside the laboratory, as in the studies presented in this book of changing quality of life (QOL) in health situations, the effective contexts for judgment are not restricted just to recent experiences. The changing context might come to include the possibility, repeatedly experienced in the imagination, that things could have been much worse. Or perhaps it is not a change in a prior context but rather a shift to a different context on a different dimension of judgment. For example, instead of judging degree of pain, the patient is now expressing a judgment on the dimension of meaningfulness: "I know that my tumor has not really grown any smaller, but I am looking at it differently now; and because I see it as a challenge to concentrate on what is meaningful, my life has actually become more meaningful." This improvement suggests that the patient's current psychological state is higher in the context of experiences judged for meaningfulness than in the context of experiences judged for painfulness.

Contemporary Applications

Because such different kinds of response shift are so evident in the field of health, it is important to be explicit about how the term is being used in each application. Any change in internalized standards for judging health can be expressed by a shift in judgment of unchanging conditions of health or by rigidity of judgment in the face of changing conditions. As defined by Sprangers and Schwartz (chapter 2), response shifts may also reflect changes in the relative weighting of different attributes of whatever condition is being judged and also changes in the conceptualization of health and thus the dimension of judgment.

In this book, the response is usually a dimensional judgment, often expressed as a self-report on some aspect of QOL within the domain of health. This kind of self-report may be in the form of a number or its associated category on a rating scale (e.g., 4 = *slightly dissatisfied* or 8 = *very satisfied*). External recalibrations of the scale that do not reflect how changes in different conditions are experienced are not response shifts in the present use of the term. For example, a rating of 4 signifies the same degree of satisfaction on a 5-point scale as a rating of 7 does on a 9-point scale. More generally, when the same set of stimuli is rated by different participants who have freely generated their own sets of rating categories, the resulting scales of judgment turn out to be linearly related (Parducci & Wedell, 1986, Experiment 1), implying that the underlying contextual effects are independent of how study participants calibrate their scales. In such cases, the researcher can easily correct for differences in scale calibration.

Any changes in response that did not reflect changes in experience would typically be of lesser interest, evidence of a response bias that must be overcome to get at what the patient is actually experiencing. Patients may report feeling better because they do, indeed, feel better; however, their reports may instead reflect their desire to please the investigator or provider. Much of the extensive literature on self-avowals of happiness seems to be subject to a bias toward reporting oneself happier than one believes most other people to be. However, we must not let either our skepticism or our search for constancies obscure real changes that might be occurring. Indeed, particularly in the area of health, an important objective of therapy may be to facilitate changes in the way particular states are experienced, changes not only in standards but also in values and conceptualizations. This is the guiding principle underlying the various contributions to this book.

As used to explain response shifts, the conception of context can be broad enough to include goals, expectations, social comparisons, counterfactual fantasies, and a number of other subjective experiences that can be represented quantitatively along with what is being judged, all on a single underlying dimension. Given the distribution of contextual values, the judgment of any particular event is strictly determined.

However, when it comes to understanding how changes in goals can be effected, contextual theory does not in itself provide answers. Nor does it deal with changes in the weightings of different attributes of whatever is being judged. It is response shift theory that calls our attention to these important considerations. To study them better, response shift theory has stimulated the development of promising new measures, such as the retrospective pretest–posttest designs (e.g., Howard et al., 1979; see also Sprangers & Hoogstraten, 1989).

This introduction has reviewed how the concept of response shift fits into the long history of judgmental relativity. Most people, even without formal training in the social sciences, would give lip service to this kind of relativism. However, it is easier to recognize the central importance of the concept of response shift than to apply it to practical effect. This book

illustrates how the concept can be applied to a wide variety of problems in the area of health, stimulating further thought and research about how standards, values, and conceptualizations change.

References

Anderson, N. A. (1981). *Foundations of information integration theory.* New York: Academic Press.

Birnbaum, M. H. (1982). Controversies in psychological measurement. In B. Wegener (Ed.), *Social attitudes and psychophysical measurement* (pp. 401–485). Hillsdale, NJ: Erlbaum.

Green, D. M., & Swets, J. A. (1966). *Signal detection theory and psychophysics.* New York: Wiley.

Helson, H. (1964). *Adaptation-level theory.* New York: Harper & Row.

Howard, G. S., Ralph, K. M., Gulanick, N. A., Maxwell, S. E., Nance, D. E., & Gerber, S. K. (1979). Internal invalidity in pretest–posttest self-report evaluations and a re-evaluation of retrospective pretests. *Applied Psychological Measurement, 3,* 1–23.

Parducci, A. (1995). *Happiness, pleasure, and judgment: The contextual theory and its applications.* Mahwah, NJ: Erlbaum.

Parducci, A., & Wedell, D. H. (1986). The category effect with rating scales: Number of categories, number of stimuli, and method of presentation. *Journal of Experimental Psychology: Human Perception and Performance, 12,* 496–516.

Sprangers, M. A. G., & Hoogstraten, J. (1989). Pretesting effects in retrospective pretest–posttest designs. *Journal of Applied Psychology, 74,* 265–272.

Torgerson, W. S. (1958). *Theory and methods of scaling.* New York: Wiley.

Wallach, H. (1948). Brightness constancy and the nature of achromatic colors. *Journal of Experimental Psychology, 38,* 310–324.

Part I

Theoretical Reflections

1

Integrating Response Shift Into Health-Related Quality-of-Life Research: A Theoretical Model

Mirjam A. G. Sprangers and Carolyn E. Schwartz

Introduction

An orthopaedic surgeon once commented that it must be difficult to study quality of life (QOL) since it not only means different things to different people, but can also mean different things to the same person over a disease trajectory. He recounts the story of a woman who, after hearing her diagnosis of osteosarcoma, told him that if her bone tumor prevented her from being able to walk, life would no longer be meaningful to her and she would prefer euthanasia. When the time came that this woman was confined to a wheelchair, she informed him that life still held value for her but that if she were to become incontinent or bedridden, then life would lose its meaning and she would prefer euthanasia. However, when the time came that she was incontinent and bedridden, the woman stated vehemently that life still held meaning for her and that she was not ready for euthanasia. This story illustrates how internal standards, values and the conceptualization of life quality can change over the course of the disease trajectory and that these changes may be inherent to the process of accommodating the illness.

This patient has undergone what is called 'response shift.' The work-

---

We would like to acknowledge the invaluable contribution of the following social and medical scientists who participated in the Response Shift Workshop held in Boston, December 1996 and funded by AHCPR (grant No. 1 RO1 HSO8582-01A1) to Dr. Schwartz and matched by a contribution from Frontier Science and Technology Research Foundation, Inc. These participants included: Achilles A. Armenakis, PhD; Katy Benjamin, SM, MSW; Lawren H. Daltroy, PhD, PH; Susan Folkman, PhD; Maureen Genderson, MA; Rick Gibbons, PhD; Hanneke C. J. M. de Haes, PhD; Hang Lee, PhD; Geraldine V. Padilla, PhD; Allen Parducci, PhD; Bruce Rapkin, PhD; Patricia Rieker, PhD; Rabbi Meir Sendor, PhD; and Ira Wilson, MD, MSc. The first author is also indebted to Frits van Dam, PhD, Hanneke de Haes, PhD, Joost Heijink, PhD, and Florence van Zuuren, PhD for stimulating discussions about response shift. We would also like to thank Florence van Zuuren for her comments on an earlier draft of this paper.

ing definition of response shift, adopted in this paper, refers to a change in the meaning of one's self-evaluation of a target construct as a result of: (a) a change in the respondent's internal standards of measurement (scale recalibration, in psychometric terms); (b) a change in the respondent's values (i.e. the importance of component domains constituting the target construct); or (c) a redefinition of the target construct (i.e. reconceptualization) (see also Schwartz & Sprangers, 1999).

Whereas the previous story is anecdotal, there is ample evidence of paradoxical and counter-intuitive findings in the literature which can be interpreted in terms of response shift. For example, patients with a life-threatening disease or disability were found to report a stable QOL (Andrykowski et al., 1993; Bach & Tilton, 1994). Moreover, a number of researchers have documented that people with a severe chronic illness report a level of QOL neither inferior nor better than that of less severely ill patients or healthy people (Cassileth et al., 1984; Stensman, 1985; Breetvelt & Van Dam, 1991; Andrykowski et al., 1993; Groenvold et al., 1999). Additionally, health care providers and significant others tend to underestimate patients' QOL as compared to patients' evaluations of their own QOL (Sprangers & Aaronson, 1992; Friedland et al., 1996; Sneeuw et al., 1996). Furthermore, cancer patients are more willing to undergo risky and toxic treatments with minimal chance of benefit than healthy people or people with a benign disease (Llewellyn-Thomas et al., 1989; O'Connor, 1989; Slevin et al., 1990), indicating that patients may have lowered their standards of tolerance and/or changed their values. Perhaps most profound is the discrepancy between clinical measures of health and patients' own evaluations of their health (Daltroy, 1999; Padilla et al., 1992; Kagawa-Singer, 1993). All of these lines of evidence suggest that response shift plays an important yet not explicitly measured role in assimilating illness.

The concept of response shift has its foundation in research on educational training interventions (Howard et al., 1979b) and organizational change (Golembiewski et al., 1976). Whereas Howard and colleagues defined response shift in terms of changes in internal standards of measurement, Golembiewski and colleagues introduced the component of reconceptualization in addition to this scale recalibration. While changes in values are inherent in Golembiewski's description of reconceptualization, the working definition adopted in this paper includes this as a separate third component that is relevant to the change in the meaning of one's self-evaluation. Making it a distinct third aspect will thus highlight its importance and emphasizes the need to measure it carefully.

The extent to which the three components of response shift are distinct or interconnected is still unknown. It may be the case that these aspects of response shift are ineluctably intertwined. Alternatively, changes in internal standards, values or conceptualization may only reflect response shift when they occur in pairs. For example, changes in internal standards may only reflect response shift when they are coincident with changes in values or changes in conceptualization. The interconnection may also reflect a hierarchical nature. For example, Golembiewski and

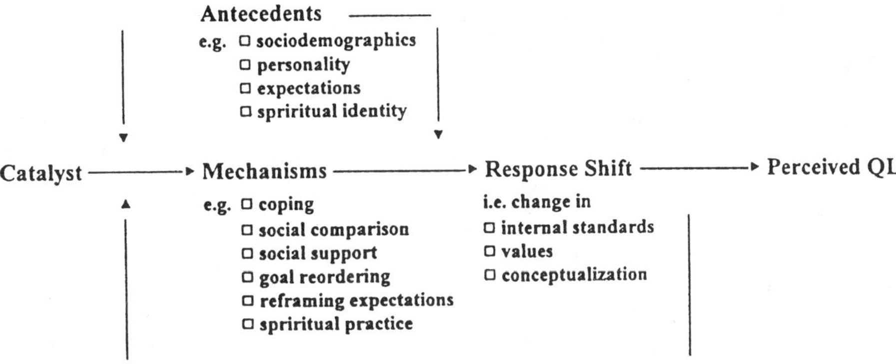

Figure 1.1. A theoretical model of response shift and quality of life (QOL).

colleagues adopted the following hierarchy, where reconceptualization needs to be ruled out before changes in internal standards can be detected. This approach makes sense since changes in internal standards of measurement will have lost their meaning if the construct itself has changed over time. Conversely, it is difficult to imagine that changes in internal standards might occur without affecting the conceptualization of the construct. Thus, while clearly distinguishing the three aspects of response shift is needed to elucidate the concept, recognizing their interconnectedness is also necessary to acknowledge the complexity and richness of the phenomenon (see also Schwartz & Sprangers, 1999).

Since response shift refers to a change in the meaning of one's self-evaluation, it may occur in any field where self-reports are required (Howard et al., 1979b). The focus of this paper will be on response shifts that may take place in the area of health-related QOL, as a result of changes in health status. Integrating response shift into health-related QOL research would enhance the sensitivity and relevance of this line of research. Understanding response shift requires a sound theoretical model. In this paper, a theoretical model is proposed to clarify and predict the occurrence or absence of response shift effects and how response shift may affect perceived QOL (Fig. 1.1). Additionally, future research directions are outlined that may further the investigation of the response shift phenomenon, by testing specific hypotheses and predictions about the QOL domains and the clinical and psychosocial conditions that may yield response shift effects.

Theoretical Model

The proposed model addresses how response shift may affect health-related QOL as a result of changes in health status. It has five major components: (1) a catalyst, (2) antecedents, (3) mechanisms, (4) response shift and (5) perceived QOL. The *catalyst* in QOL research would refer to a change in the respondent's health status, that may or may not result from a treatment. The *antecedents* refer to stable or dispositional characteristics of the individual. Examples of such antecedents include sociodemographics (e.g. gender, education) and personality (e.g. optimism, self-esteem, sense of control, mastery) (Ormel, 1983; Costa & McCrae, 1980; De Haes, 1988; Scheier et al., 1989), expectations (Scheier & Carver, 1987), or spiritual identity. *Mechanisms* will refer to behavioral, cognitive, and affective processes to accommodate the catalyst. Examples of such mechanisms include using coping strategies (Lazarus & Folkman, 1984; Folkman, 1997); initiating social comparisons (Taylor & Lobel, 1989; Van Der Zee et al., 1995; Gibbons, 1999); seeking social support (Cohen & Wills, 1985; Sarason et al., 1985; Taylor et al., 1986); reordering goals (Rapkin & Fischer, 1992); reframing expectations (Heyink, 1993; Allison et al., 1997) and engaging in spiritual practice (Park et al., 1990; Koenig, 1997; Richards & Folkman, 1997). The working definition of *response shift* is a change in the meaning of one's self-evaluation of QOL as a result of changes in internal standards, values and the conceptualization of QOL. *Perceived QOL* may be defined as a multidimensional construct incorporating at least three broad domains—physical, psychological and social functioning (Siegrist & Junge, 1989; Cella & Tulsky, 1990; McMillen Moinpour et al., 1990). Beyond this core set of QOL domains, additional issues may be more salient for some individuals (e.g. spirituality and intimacy) or more relevant for specific patient groups depending on the functional domains affected by the disease (e.g. sexuality and body image).

Changes in an individual's health status may prompt behavioral, cognitive and affective processes necessary for accommodating illness. These processes have the potential to change an individual's standards, values or conceptualization of QOL and this response shift will thus influence perceived QOL. The kind of mechanisms that an individual will engage in as well as the magnitude and type of the resulting response shift (i.e. changes in standards, values or conceptualization) will be dependent on dispositional characteristics. Thus, the antecedents are postulated to have both indirect and direct effects on potentiating response shift. Perceiving a suboptimal QOL may lead the individual to reinitiate established or new mechanisms. This feedback loop is aimed at maintaining or improving the perception of QOL. Clearly, this process is iterative and dynamic by definition.

Illustration

Three examples are provided to elucidate this preliminary model. Imagine three women, Jane, Ann and Mary, all of whom are diagnosed with Stage 3 breast cancer. Jane expects that she is able to control important features of her day-to-day life, and thus has a generalized expectancy of an internal locus of control. When confronted with her diagnosis, Jane would seek to maintain a sense of control. However, her focus remains on controlling disease-specific domains which are not currently within her control. Consequently, she experiences frequent episodes of helplessness, frustration, and depression because she is not able to accomplish her usual level of work and other activities. Jane's behavior is not likely to result in response shift because she has not changed her internal standards, has not changed her values, nor has she reconceptualized QOL. Consequently, her perceived QOL will be worse than her QOL prior to diagnosis.

In contrast to Jane, Ann has the tendency to expect that powerful others exert control over her day-to-day life. When confronted with her diagnosis, she would seek to engage in spiritual practice that might include prayer and reading religious texts. She might engage in downward social comparison, by talking with and supporting less fortunate other people with a similar diagnosis. These behaviors might induce response shift due to changes in *internal standards*, since her idea of poor functioning may now be anchored at a much lower level than previously conceived. Additionally, by engaging in spiritual practice and by developing a role of helping other people whose conditions are worse, she may create a new sense of purpose in life which may modify her *conceptualization of QOL*. Thus, Ann might experience a similar level of QOL to that experienced prior to diagnosis.

Like Jane, and in contrast to Ann, Mary has always tended to perceive herself as being able to control important features of her day-to-day life. When confronted with this diagnosis, she would seek to maintain an internal sense of control by reordering her goals and engaging in upward social comparison. For example, since health is no longer controllable to her and her energy level may not allow her to work as she used to, she might focus her attention on developing more intimate family relationships rather than professional accomplishments, which had been her focus prior to diagnosis. She might also seek positive role models, such as women who have succeeded in overcoming a similar disease. These behaviors may induce response shift that results in the first place from changes in *values*, i.e. in the relative importance of QOL domains as family life gained in importance relative to a professional career. Additionally, by changing her focus to other role models, she might perceive overcoming the disease as within her power, and might develop an appreciation of her social and emotional resources (Bach & Tilton, 1994). This appreciation might result in a change in her *conceptualization of QOL*. Thus Mary might experience a level of QOL similar to or better than one which she had experienced prior to diagnosis.

In these three examples, the antecedents and mechanisms are differentially effective in inducing response shift, and consequently in reducing, maintaining or improving QOL. These examples also illustrate that this process can implicate more than one aspect of response shift. For the sake of simplicity, we have used only a limited number of antecedents and mechanisms, but this is not to imply that only one or two of these variables should be considered in modeling response shift.

Discussion of the Model

Conceiving the proposed model as a single process would be overly simplistic and would do injustice to the complex, multifaceted, and dynamic reality of psychological adaptation to illness. Rather, the model is meant as a framework which may guide the conceptualization and measurement (Schwartz & Sprangers, 1999) of QOL over time. Additionally, this model is not new from clinical (Wilson, 1999) or theoretical perspectives. For example, it has similarities with control theory's approach to the understanding of self-regulating systems. The central aspect of control theory is the feed-back loop aimed at reducing sensed discrepancies from a comparison value to explain how people maintain an acceptable level of health, well-being or any other self-definition (Powers, 1978; Carver & Scheier, 1982; Leventhal & Nerenz, 1983). The proposed model is not meant to replace such or other (derived) theories that purport to explain health-related QOL, including adaptation theories (Helson, 1964; Brickman & Campbell, 1971; Taylor, 1983; Parducci, 1995), discrepancy theories (Calman, 1984; Michalos, 1985), uncertainty in illness theory (Mishel, 1988, 1990; Padilla et al., 1992), or stress-coping theories (Lazarus & Folkman, 1984). Rather, to the extent that response shift is demonstrated to have explanatory power, its incorporation is recommended in such existing theories. While all these theories make important and convincing attempts to explain perceived well-being from different angles and with different foci, none of them takes response shift explicitly into account.

The strength of including response shift is first that it conceptualizes three salient aspects of change. Making these aspects explicit in the model will allow a better understanding of how QOL is affected by changes in health status, as well as by medical or psychosocial interventions. Second, elucidating these aspects will direct the development of reliable and valid measures for assessing change in QOL (see Schwartz & Sprangers, 1999).

For example, according to the cognitive theory of stress and coping (Lazarus & Folkman, 1984) and its recent modification (Folkman, 1997), people are constantly appraising their interactions with their environment. Interactions that are appraised as stressful (e.g. a cancer diagnosis) require coping to accommodate the stressor. Coping processes lead to an event outcome which may be positive, negative or may not yield a resolution. Emotion is generated throughout the processes of appraisal, coping and event outcomes. This model may gain in explanatory power when response shift is postulated prior to event and emotional outcomes, thus rendering it consistent with the proposed model. By explicitly addressing changes in internal standards, values and the conceptualization of outcome, the subtlety and complexity of the adaptation process will be more comprehensively captured.

A second example might be past research which suggests no or minimal effectiveness of a psychosocial or medical intervention on perceived QOL. If such studies were to integrate response shift in their evaluations, they might be more responsive to the full treatment impact. Indeed, response shift can be viewed as an important component of a treatment effect, or alternatively of the longitudinal trajectory of perceived QOL. It may be the case that treatments that induce a response shift are more tolerable and result in better treatment adherence than those which do not. For example, an important factor of treatment adherence might be the extent to which a medical treatment challenges values that are central to a person. To illustrate, young women with lupus, whose self-esteem is highly dependent on body image, would be less likely to be able to tolerate side effects of steroids (e.g. facial disfiguration) because they are unable to change that central value. Conversely, these same women might be better able to tolerate the comparatively severe gastro-intestinal side effects of methotrexate because their self-image is not challenged. Given their values and preferences they might be more committed to maintaining the methotrexate therapy and might consequently shift their internal standards of gastro-intestinal discomfort to maintain an acceptable level of QOL.

An initial recognition of response shift came in the context of the lack of change in perceived QOL despite clinical or objective deterioration (Andrykowski et al., 1993; Bach & Tilton, 1994). Thus, one crucial assumption of this model is that people want to feel as good as possible about themselves, either in the past or present. With its roots in control theory, response shift is thus directed toward maintaining or regaining homeostasis. The corollary assumption is that the model is dynamic. In the face of continuous change, such flexibility would be necessary to maintain or regain an acceptable perceived level of QOL. For example, if health status improves dramatically but transiently, the individual might shift his or her internal standards, values and the conceptualization of QOL to adjust to this changing level. If the individual were unable to adjust to subsequent deterioration and maintained those higher standards that were appropriate when his or her health was better, then the initial response shift becomes maladaptive. It is thus critical that the aspects of response shift be continuously and flexibly readdressed over the course of the disease trajectory.

At this early stage in model development, our understanding of the dynamics which may lead to response shift is limited to those situations where response shifts seem adaptive. Thus, our examples are teleological as we are postulating response shift as a mechanism by which perceived QOL does not deteriorate in the face of deteriorating health status. Indeed, the most obvious examples of research or anecdotal evidence are more suggestive of the adaptive than of the maladaptive potential of response shift. For example, response shift might serve as a buffer of the stressful impact of deteriorating health on psychological well-being (Schwartz et al., 1995). It is conceivable, however, that response shift would be maladaptive in some contexts. The example provided above pertained to an individual's inability to adapt adequately to changes in health status. Another example may refer to an individual who has a health condition that requires problem-focused vigilance. It would be maladaptive to change internal standards of his/her symptoms or functional limitations if this shift were to prevent him or her from utilizing appropriate health care services or treatment regimens. Furthermore, the model does not require that response shift be a conscious process. The consciousness or intentionality of response shift may differ across individuals.

Clearly, not all changes or lack of changes in QOL are driven by response shift. By definition, response shift is not at stake when patients' internal standards, values, or conceptualization of QOL remain unaffected. However, given the preliminary stage of model development and the scarcity of empirical data, the identification or prediction of the situations where response shift does not play a role is necessarily tentative. For example, one might expect that the occurrence of response shift will be less likely in areas of behavioral change, instrumental coping, and learning appropriate compensatory or preventive skills (e.g. walking with a cane, caring for a stoma, cooking according to dietary restrictions). Clearly, such activities may be of paramount importance in accommodating the illness, but may not necessarily affect the internal standards, values or conceptualization of QOL. Additionally, one might hypothesize that response tendencies such as social desirability, effort justification and cognitive dissonance reduction may induce changes in reported QOL, without actually affecting internal standards, values or the conceptualization of QOL. For example, patients with symptomatic gallstones who were randomized to either laparoscopic cholecystectomy with day care or laparoscopic cholecystectomy in the hospital, preferred retrospectively the treatment they had received, independent of the treatment actually received (Keulemans et al., 1977). This retrospective preference may be viewed as an example of cognitive dissonance reduction rather than response shift. However, such response tendencies may also potentiate response shift. For example, Diener et al. (1991) demonstrated that social desirability may not be a response artifact, but rather a personality characteristic that may help people to assimilate illness and enjoy a higher level of QOL.

Future Research Directions

There are many aspects of this theoretical model that need to be developed in future research. The components of the model, including the catalyst, antecedents, mechanisms and perceived QOL, would benefit from investigations which highlight or identify the specific conditions which would potentiate or prevent response shifts. Regarding the *catalyst*, it would be important to identify what parameters of health state changes or interventions would initiate the response shift process. Parameters that would merit attention include the rate of onset of the health status change (i.e. sudden or gradual), its duration, severity, pervasiveness and direction (i.e. improvement or deterioration). Finally, it is conceivable that response shifts occur merely with the passage of time, without clear changes in health status and/or the underlying pathology. Time does change patients, if only because there is a longer past with disease and a greater number of experiences that occur in the interim that may affect internal standards, values, and the conceptualization of life quality. Thus, an additional question is related to the extent that response shift may be elicited by the mere passage of time or by entering new developmental stages in life (Erikson, 1963).

Regarding the *antecedents*, research is needed to address which dispositional characteristics play a role in the response shift process. For example, personality characteristics such as self-esteem or optimism might promote response shift, while depression or locus of control might impede it. Additionally, people may have different thresholds for recognizing or tolerating health status change, an extreme example of a low threshold being somatization disorder. The characteristic feature of somatization is the rigidity by which these patients conceptualize their symptoms and their resistance to efforts to change these dysfunctional cognitions (Wilson, 1999). Alternatively, people with a high level of tolerance for symptoms, may not feel the need to engage in adaptive strategies. Consequently, both people with lower or higher thresholds are hypothesized to be less inclined to undergo response shifts, albeit for different reasons. Additionally, future research should examine whether different characteristics are implicated at different stages of the disease trajectory. For example, one might hypothesize that sociodemographic factors might be implicated early on and that different personality characteristics might play a significant role at subsequent phases of the disease trajectory. The rationale for this hypothesis is that sociodemographic characteristics, such as gender, age, level of education and ethnic background may affect early presentation of symptoms (i.e. patient's delay). Personality characteristics, such as optimism and mastery, are related to coping mechanisms (Pearlin & Schooler, 1978; Scheier & Carver, 1987) and by definition may play a role at a later stage in the disease trajectory.

With respect to the *mechanisms*, research is needed that will clarify how these mechanisms relate to response shift, how they relate to each other, how they are moderated by the antecedents, and how they may be influenced by the illness trajectory. For example, since it is easier to change one's cognition (e.g. aspiration level) than affect (e.g. emotional well-being) (Campbell et al., 1976, De Haes et al., 1992), it is hypothesized that in early stages of the disease trajectory cognitive coping strategies will be initiated, while emotion-focused coping will be adopted later on. This model would be best served by empirically examining the interrelationships and feedback loops. Subsequent work might then enumerate additional mechanisms.

With respect to *perceived QOL*, response shift is expected to be more prevalent in domains which are more cognitive (e.g. satisfaction, achievement of life goals and cognitive ability) rather than affective (e.g. emotional well-being, mood and distress) (Campbell et al., 1976, De Haes et al., 1992). Additionally, one might hypothesize that response shift is more likely to occur in those domains which are subjective (e.g. pain, fatigue and interpersonal relationships) rather than objective (e.g. physical functioning, role performance and work disability). While one might predict that response shift would occur in more global assessments of QOL domains, future research should evaluate whether specific assessments of the same QOL domains will reveal comparable response shift effects. Similarly, behaviorally-anchored items might be less prone to response shift than affectively- or cognitively-worded items, although research in educational interventions found response shift effects in both types of questions (Howard et al., 1979a).

While the proposed model postulates a dynamic *feedback loop*, investigating this process is complicated by time-dependent parameters that are currently undefined. For example, it is unknown how long it takes for response shifts to occur. Thus accurately tracking this process will be facilitated when the desired interval for data collection is known.

While all of the above components merit considerable investigation, perhaps the most fundamental work on response shift is related to broader questions about the overall significance of this model. Specifically, the contribution of response shift to QOL research will depend on whether it increases the explained variance in both objective health status and subjective well-being measures (see Daltroy et al., 1999). Additionally, its contribution would be supported if it facilitates better prediction of future QOL. Of related importance would be investigations which clarify which aspects of response shift highlight or attenuate longitudinal or intervention effects. For example, interventions aimed at changing cognitions (e.g. aspiration level) might induce changes in internal standards of measurement, while interventions focusing on affect (e.g. psychological well-being) might result in changes in values and the conceptualization of QOL. Additionally, stress-management interventions as well as effective doctor–patient communication may actually 'teach' response shifts by training people to change their internal standards, values or the conceptualization of QOL.

This complex unfolding might well be investigated in longitudinal research with multiple time points, incorporating standardized assessments of selected antecedents, mechanisms and perceived QOL, as well as additional measures of response shift (see Schwartz & Sprangers, 1999). To capture fully the impact of response shift in QOL research, such investigations should preferably be conducted in a large range of acutely and chronically ill patients whose illness differs in stage, severity and pervasiveness. Revealing the full impact of response shift may be critical for research which aims to evaluate QOL over time in observational studies comparing different patient groups, or in intervention studies of adaptation to illness.

References

Allison, P. J., Locker, D., & Feine, J. S. (1997). Quality of life: A dynamic construct. *Social Science & Medicine, 45,* 221–230.

Andrykowski, M. A., Brady, M. J., & Hunt, J. W. (1993). Positive psychosocial adjustment in potential bone marrow transplant recipients: Cancer as a psychosocial transition. *Psycho-Oncology, 2,* 261–276.

Bach, J. R., & Tilton, M. C. (1994). Life satisfaction and well-being measures in ventilator assisted individuals with traumatic tetraplegia. *Archives Phys. Med. Rehabilitation, 75,* 626–632.

Breetvelt, I. S., & Van Dam, F. S. A. M. (1991). Underreporting by cancer patients: The case of response shift. *Social Science & Medicine, 32,* 981–987.

Brickman, P., & Campbell, D. T. (1971). Hedonic relativism and planning the good society. In M. H. Appley (Ed.), *Adaptation level theory: A symposium.* New York: Academic Press.
Calman, K. C. (1984). Quality of life in cancer patients: An hypothesis. *Journal of Medical Ethics, 10,* 124–127.
Campbell, A., Converse, P. E., & Rodgers, W. L. (1976). *The quality of American life.* New York: Sage.
Carver, C. S., & Scheier, M. F. (1982). Control theory: A useful conceptual framework for personality, social, clinical, and health psychology. *Psychological Bulletin, 92,* 111–135.
Cassileth, B. R., Lusk, E. J., & Tenaglia, A. N. (1984). A psychological comparison of patients with melanoma and other dermatological disorders. *American Academy of Dermatology, 7,* 742–746.
Cella, D. F., & Tulsky, D. S. (1990). Measuring quality of life today: Methodological aspects. *Oncology, 4,* 29–38.
Cohen, S., & Wills, T. A. (1985). Stress, social support, and the buffering hypothesis. *Psychological Bulletin, 98,* 310–357.
Costa, P. T., & McCrae, R. R. (1980). Influence of extraversion and neuroticism on subjective well-being: Happy and unhappy people. *Journal of Personality and Social Psychology, 38,* 668–678.
Daltroy, L. H., Larson, M. G., Eaton, H. M., Phillips, C. B., & Liang, M. H. (1999). Discrepancies between self-reported and observed physical function in the elderly: The influence of response shift and other factors. *Social Science & Medicine, 48,* 1549–1562.
De Haes, J. C. J. M. (1988). Kwaliteit van leven van kankerpatiënten. Dissertation. Swets & Zeitlinger, Lisse.
De Haes, J. C. J. M., De Ruiter, J. H., Tempelaar, R., & Pennink, B. J. W. (1992). The distinction between affect and cognition in the quality of life of cancer patients: Sensitivity and stability. *Quality of Life Research, 1,* 315–322.
Diener, E., Sandvik, E., Pavot, W., & Gallagher, D. (1991). Response artifacts in the measurement of subjective well-being. *Social Indicators Research, 24,* 35–56.
Erikson, E. (1963). *Childhood and society.* New York: Norton.
Folkman, S. (1997). Positive psychological states and coping with severe stress. *Social Science & Medicine, 45,* 1207–1221.
Friedland, J., Renwick, R., & McColl, M. (1996). Coping and social support as determinants of quality of life in HIV/AIDS. *AIDS Care, 8,* 15–31.
Gibbons, F. X. (1999). Social Comparison as a mediator of response shift. *Social Science & Medicine, 48,* 1517–1530.
Golembiewski, R. T., Billingsley, K., & Yeager, S. (1976). Measuring change and persistence in human affairs: Types of change generated by OD designs. *Journal of Applied Behavioral Science, 12,* 133–157.
Groenvold, M., Fayers, P. M., Sprangers, M. A. G., Bjorner, J. B., Klee, M. C., Aaronson, N. K., Bech, P., & Mouridsen, H. T. (1999). Anxiety and depression in breast cancer patients at low risk of recurrence compared with the general population: Unexpected findings. *Journal of Clinical Epidemiology, 52,* 523–530.
Helson, H. (1964). *Adaptation level theory.* New York: Harper & Row.
Heyink, J. (1993). Adaptation and well-being. *Psychological Reports, 73,* 1331–1342.
Howard, G. S., Dailey, P. R., & Gulanick, N. A. (1979a). The feasibility of informed pretests in attenuating response-shift bias. *Applied Psychological Measurement, 3,* 481–494.
Howard, G. S., Ralph, K. M., Gulanick, N. A., Maxwell, S. E., Nance, S. W., & Gerber, S. K. (1979b). Internal invalidity in pretest–posttest self-report evaluations and a reevaluation of retrospective pretests. *Applied Psychological Measurement, 3,* 1–23.
Kagawa-Singer, M. (1993). Redefining health: Living with cancer. *Social Science & Medicine, 37,* 295–304.
Keulemans, Y. C. A., Eshuis, J. H., De Haes, J. C. J. M., Leeuwenberg, A., De Wit, L. T., & Gouma, D. J. (1997). Day-care laparoscopic cholecystectomy compared to laparoscopic cholecystectomy with hospital admission (a randomized trial). In Keulemans, Y. Pathogenesis and Treatment. Dissertation, University of Amsterdam.
Koenig, H. G. (1997). Use of religion by patients with severe medical illness. *Mind/Body Medicine, 2,* 31–36.
Lazarus, R. S., & Folkman, S. (1984). *Stress, appraisal, and coping.* New York: Springer.

Leventhal, H., & Nerenz, D. R. (1983). A model for stress research with some implications for the control stress disorders. In D. Meichenbaum & M. Jaremko (Eds.), *Stress reduction and prevention* (pp. 5–38). New York: Plenum Press.

Llewellyn-Thomas, H. A., Thiel, E. C., & Clark, R. M. (1989). Patients versus surrogates: Whose opinion counts on the ethics review panels? *Clinical Research, 37,* 51–55.

McMillen Moinpour, C., Hayden, K., Thompson, I. M., et al. (1990). Quality of life assessment in southwest oncology group trials. *Oncology, 4,* 79–89.

Michalos, A. C. (1985). Multiple discrepancies theory (MDT). *Social Indicators Research, 16,* 347–413.

Mishel, M. H. (1988). Uncertainty in illness. *Journal Nursing Scholarship, 20,* 225–232.

Mishel, M. H. (1990). Reconceptualization of the uncertainty in illness theory. *Image: Journal Nursing Scholarship, 22,* 256–264.

O'Connor, A. M. (1989). Effects of framing and level of probability on patients' preferences for cancer chemotherapy. *Journal of Clinical Epidemiology, 42,* 119–126.

Ormel, J. (1983). Neuroticism and well-being inventories: Measuring traits or states? *Psychological Medicine, 13,* 165–176.

Padilla, G. V., Mishel, M. H., & Grant, M. M. (1992). Uncertainty, appraisal, and quality of life. *Quality of Life Research, 1,* 155–165.

Parducci, A. (1995). Value judgements: Happiness, pleasure, and judgment. New Jersey: Lawrence Erlbaum Associates.

Park, C., Cohen, L. H., & Herb, I. (1990). Intrinsic religiousness and religious coping as life stress moderators for Catholics versus Protestants. *Journal of Personality and Social Psychology, 59,* 562–574.

Pearlin, L. I., & Schooler, C. (1978). The structure of coping. *Journal of Health and Social Behavior, 19,* 2–21.

Powers, W. T. (1978). Quantitative analysis of purposive systems: Some spadework at the foundations of scientific psychology. *Psychological Review, 85,* 417–435.

Rapkin, B. D., & Fischer, K. (1992). Framing the construct of life satisfaction in terms of older adults' personal goals. *Psychology and Aging, 7,* 138–149.

Richards, T. A., & Folkman, S. (1997). Spiritual aspects of loss at the time of a partner's death from AIDS. *Death Studies, 21,* 527–551.

Sarason, I. G., Sarason, B. R., Potter, E. H., & Antoni, M. H. (1985). Life events, social support, and illness. *Psychosomatic Medicine, 47,* 156–163.

Scheier, M. F., & Carver, C. S. (1987). Dispositional optimism and physical well-being: The influence of generalised outcome expectancies on health. *Journal of Personality, 55,* 169–210.

Scheier, M. F., Magovern, G. J., Abbott, R. A., Matthews, K. A., Owens, J. F., Lefebvre, R. C., & Carver, C. S. (1989). Dispositional optimism and recovery from coronary artery bypass surgery: The beneficial effects on physical and psychological well-being. *Journal of Personality and Social Psychology, 57,* 1024–1040.

Schwartz, C. E., & Sprangers, M. A. G. (1999). Methodological approaches for assessing response shift in longitudinal quality of life research. *Social Science & Medicine, 48,* 1531–1548.

Schwartz, C. E., Foley, F. W., Rao, S. M., Bernardin, L. J., Lipshutz, M., & Kashala, P. (1995). A prospective study of stressful life events and course of disease in multiple sclerosis [Abstract]. *Psychometric Medicine, 57,* 89.

Siegrist, J., & Junge, A. (1989). Conceptual and methodological problems in research on the quality of life in clinical medicine. *Social Science & Medicine, 29,* 463–468.

Slevin, M. L., Stubbs, L., Plant, H. J., Wilson, P., Gregory, W. M., Armes, P. J., & Downer, S. M. (1990). Attitudes to chemotherapy: Comparing views of patients with cancer with those of doctors, nurses, and general public. *British Medical Journal, 300,* 1458–1460.

Sneeuw, K. C. A., Aaronson, N. K., Sprangers, M. A. G., Detmar, S. B., Wever, L. D. V., & Schornagel, J. H. (1996). The value of caregiver ratings in evaluating the quality of life of patients with cancer. *Journal of Clinical Oncology, 15,* 1206–1217.

Sprangers, M. A. G., & Aaronson, N. K. (1992). The role of health care providers and significant others in evaluating the quality of life of patients with chronic disease: A review. *Journal of Clinical Epidemiology, 45,* 743–760.

Stensman, R. (1985). Severely mobility-disabled people assess the quality of their lives. *Scandinavian Journal of Rehabilitation Medicine, 17,* 87–99.

Taylor, S. E. (1983). Adjustment to threatening events: A theory of cognitive adaptation. *American Psychologist, 59,* 1161–1173.

Taylor, S. E., Falke, R. L., Shoptaw, S. J., & Lichtman, R. R. (1986). Social support, support groups and the cancer patient. *Journal of Consulting and Clinical Psychology, 54,* 608–615.

Taylor, S. E., & Lobel, M. (1989). Social comparison activity under threat: Downward evaluation and upward contacts. *Psychological Reviews, 96,* 569–575.

Van Der Zee, K. I., Buunk, B. P., & Sanderman, R. (1995). Social comparison as a mediator between health problems and subjective health evaluations. *British Journal of Social Psychology, 34,* 53–65.

Wilson, I. B. (1999). Clinical understanding and clinical implications of response shift. *Social Science & Medicine, 48,* 1577–1588.

2

Response Shift: A Coping Perspective

T. Anne Richards and Susan Folkman

Response shift refers to changes in internal standards, values, and conceptualization of quality of life (QOL; see chapters 1 and 6). This book focuses on response shifts that may occur as a result of changes in health status that is improving or deteriorating. Although response shift does not always have positive effects on the experience of life quality, there can occur a change that causes an enhancement of the experience of daily living, despite worsening conditions. This interpretation helps explain findings from studies suggesting that people subjectively experience a QOL that seems incongruent with the observable circumstances (Andrykowski, Brady, & Hunt, 1993; Breetvelt & van Dam, 1991; Frankl, 1959).

Our understanding of response shift draws on principles of adaptive coping (Folkman & Stein, 1996). According to these principles, an individual must first be able to relinquish unrealistic beliefs about how things are; revise those beliefs; and then substitute new, downwardly revised expectations that are consistent with the revised beliefs. Second, the individual must be able to attach positive value and meaning to the new expectations. This process may involve revising core beliefs about the self and about what is valued and meaningful. The process depends on the activation of a particular class of coping processes, namely, meaning-based coping. In this chapter we present a framework with which to specify coping mechanisms that can create and sustain the phenomenon of response shift.

We consider response shift in the context of a study of caregiving for a partner dying of AIDS and the subsequent experience of bereavement —a context characterized by deterioration of the most profound sort. Although our research focused on coping (i.e., we did not intend to explore the concept of response shift in these caregivers), we found that caregivers were able to maintain impressive levels of positive psychological well-being despite the deteriorating and stressful circumstances of their partners' disease progression and death and their own high levels of concomitant distress. As a consequence, we have extensive data that may provide

---

Work on this chapter was supported by National Institute of Mental Health Grants MH49985 and MH52517 awarded to Susan Folkman, PI.

some insight into the phenomenon of response shift in terms of how it comes about and how it is maintained. We begin by briefly describing the study and the empirical data that is consistent with the notion of response shift. We will use qualitative data that illustrate the processes through which response shift is achieved and maintained through the principles of adaptive coping.

University of California, San Francisco, Coping Project

The University of California, San Francisco (UCSF) Coping Project was a longitudinal study of caregiving and bereavement among partners of men with AIDS, which was conducted in the San Francisco area from 1990 to 1997. Participants were gay men who were primary caregivers for partners diagnosed with AIDS. The average length of relationship at entry to the study was slightly more than six years. One third of the caregiving partners were themselves infected with HIV. Inclusion criteria required participants to be healthy (have no more than two symptoms of HIV) at the time of enrollment. Initially, 253 caregivers enrolled and were followed for two years. At the end of two years, 195 participants agreed to continue for an additional three years; 145 participants completed the study, for a total of five years. During the course of the two phases of the study, 158 men were bereaved. Attrition was due to dropout, illness, and death.

Participants were assessed bimonthly during the first two years and biannually during the next three years on their moods, life stressors, social support, coping processes, and physical health. They also had semiannual physical exams and mental health assessments. Qualitative data were collected through semistructured and open-ended interviews bimonthly, biannually, at the time of bereavement, and on exit from the study.

Marking Loss

Our study was conducted before protease inhibitors and other highly reactive antiviral treatments were available; caring for a partner with AIDS was typically a long and arduous process (Folkman, Chesney, & Christopher-Richards, 1994). The disease course was uneven and unpredictable, and the opportunistic infections that punctuated the process were usually clinically complex and frequently horrific. Over the course of the disease, the caregiver needed to adjust to changes, usually for the worse, in his partner's physical and emotional health, which typically involved acknowledging loss.

To the casual observer, some losses might seem trivial. For example, social engagements often had to be limited, excursions had to be scheduled for shorter periods, and more of the housework may have had to be shifted to the caregiver. But such losses signaled meaningful changes in the relationship between the caregiver and his partner. For example, changes in social life could lead to a loss of shared laughter and intimacy that simple enjoyments provide. The shift in responsibility often signaled the decline of the partner's autonomy and dependence on the caregiver. Decline in health frequently carried with it the loss of sexual intimacy.

Many caregivers grieved these losses and talked openly about them in their narratives. The grieving of day-to-day losses is part of the process of giving up expectations that are no longer realistic, which we hold as a necessary process if a response shift is to occur. Said one participant, "I'm losing him in bits and pieces. It's not like he's hit by a car and then gone. I lose him a little at a time, it's excruciating" (Folkman et al., 1994, p. 43).

Developing New Expectations and Discovering Their Positive Meanings

The caregivers in this study were for the most part realistic about what was happening to their partners. Expectations for growing old together were abandoned, as were more immediate expectations for companionship and intimacy. New expectations evolved; the most pervasive was the expectation that caregiving would take up the next months and possibly even years.

Earlier we stated that for a response shift to occur, new expectations had to be valued and meaningful. Meaning is found or created by accessing beliefs and values. Some of these beliefs and values were relevant only to the immediate situation, whereas others touched on deeply held core beliefs that were central to the person's definition of himself (cf. Park & Folkman, 1997). We have chosen to focus on the caregiving role to illustrate the processes through which caregivers found positive meaning in the deteriorating circumstances of their partner's decline.

Our interviews initially focused on the stressful aspects of caregiving. Early in the study several participants complained that by asking only about the stressful aspects of caregiving, we were getting a biased portrait of their lives. They said we should be asking about the positive meanings of caregiving. We took their advice, and as a consequence we found substantial evidence in both the quantitative and qualitative data of the meaning-making process. We constructed a scale that described benefits that can be derived from caregiving (Folkman, Chesney, Collette, Boccellari, & Cooke, 1996). The scale included items such as "Caregiving makes me feel needed," "Caregiving shows my love for my partner," and "Caregiving has brought me closer to my partner." The men's responses to this questionnaire were markedly positive. More than 85% agreed or strongly agreed with 5 of the 6 of the items. Clearly, these sources of meaning were relevant in caregivers' lives.

Perhaps the most compelling accounts of the positive meaning of caregiving came from narratives in which caregivers were describing stressful events related to their caregiving. We find it noteworthy that these were unsolicited comments about the positive meanings of caregiving that were provided in the context of a stressful event. Sometimes the meaning was specific to the situation that was being described, as in the following example:

> He is having neuropathy. The other night I was home and his feet were bothering him and his toes were very sensitive. We were alone. He was in bed. I did some Reiki (energy transference) on his feet. It wasn't upsetting to me. It was something that happened and I did the best I could. It was acceptance. I'm qualified in Reiki and I did it. It felt good. If anything, it had the opposite effect, it was a way of being closer. I felt grateful that there was something I could do to comfort him.

Other times, the caregiver recognized that the meaning touched on deeply held values and beliefs and was central to his definition of self:

> The creation of something has always been a favorite accomplishment and doing a project together, we are always at our best. My willingness to jump into this project has been a much better response than what my friends said to do. I could have stopped this. Fear could have stopped this. So many of my friends say no to their lovers out of fear that what they do might make them more sick. I did the opposite instinctively. I encouraged him and I know that I could have put an end to all of this. The glass is always half full and that's what you work with. Encouraging your own and someone else's creativity is life-giving.

Finding Meaning in the Ordinary

Meaning that contributed to the caregiver's QOL was also derived from everyday events of life that were often unrelated to caregiving (Folkman, Moskowitz, Ozer, & Park, 1997). Positive meaningful events were reported in 99.5% of 1,794 interviews. When asked, caregivers had little difficulty recalling and describing simple events that enhanced their daily experience. In analyzing 215 events of 36 participants over a one-year period, we found that these were ordinary events that brought fulfillment and meaning into the caregivers' lives. Events most frequently were related to social occasions, entertainment, meaningful conversations, or work. The events provided feelings of connection and being cared for, feelings of a sense of achievement and self-esteem, or feelings of respite from everyday affairs. For example, one participant said, "Tim bought me a card. It let me know his feelings are there, and as strong as mine are. And that he was thinking about me enough to buy a card and give it." Another participant stated,

> We went to a double bill at the Castro [a movie theater] on Sunday. It was *The Women* and *All About Eve*. I recited all the lines from *The Women* and Brad recited all the lines from *All About Eve*, and we screamed and laughed for three hours. We had a blast. It was a shared experience, something we knew we'd both enjoy. I was very happy, very much a part of a community.

Half of the meaningful events were planned and half occurred spontaneously. It is possible that these ordinary events took on additional significance because they were situated in the stressful circumstances of caregiving. In a less stressful environment, the events may have held a different meaning. In this sense, the events held situational meaning and were not as deeply tied to the caregiver's core beliefs about self and the world-at-large compared to the self-defining meaning we described earlier.

Distinguishing General Versus Situational Meaning

The two kinds of meaning that we have described—the meaning attached to caregiving and the meaning attached to the ordinary events of day-to-day life—refer to two levels of meaning. Global meaning is built on beliefs that are stable and central to the individual's understanding of the self and the self's relationship to the world. The kind of meaning that is derived from ordinary day-to-day events is more likely to be situational. Situational meaning is built on beliefs that are not necessarily stable or core. Because situational meaning is less deeply rooted, less generalized, and less stable than global meaning, it is more easily modifiable (Park & Folkman, 1997). The meaning associated with caregiving is more likely to be global, touching on deeply held core values and beliefs, and the meaning associated with the ordinary events of daily life is more likely to be situational.

Both global and situational meaning have important roles in sustaining a response shift. Sprangers and Schwartz (chapter 1) referred to an internal recalibration that occurs in which standards for a QOL shift in some way in response to the changing circumstances. We speculate that if a recalibration occurs, it will be at the level of global meaning. As global meanings shift, the assumptive world is altered so that a redefinition of self and place in the world occurs. It would then follow that situational meanings alter in response to the shift in core beliefs. Concordance of situational and global meaning is achieved, and this helps support the recalibration.

Reinforcing Response Shift Through Meaning and Goal Process

Meaning helps motivate the individual to formulate goals; it provides direction and purpose (Antonovsky, 1987; Baumeister, 1991; Csikszentmihalyi, 1990; Emmons & Kaiser, 1996; Reker & Wong, 1988). Stein, Folkman, Trabasso, and Richards (1997) defined *goals* as "imaginable states of existence that are desired, and refer to any valued object, activity, or state that a person wants to attain" (p. 873). When people formulate goals, they often create plans with which to achieve those goals. These plans and goals direct the individual to active, problem-focused forms of coping (for a review, see Carver & Scheier, 1998).

Goals, plans, and problem-focused coping can play an important role in response shift. People formulate goals based in part on their beliefs and expectations. To the extent that a response shift involves a downward revision of expectations, so, too, goals must be revised and reformulated to match the new reality (Folkman & Stein, 1996; Stein et al., 1997). To the extent that the person makes successful progress toward, or achievement of, such goals, he or she will experience positive well-being (Carver & Scheier, 1998), which in turn provides important reinforcement for the response shift.

Just as we discussed meaning at global and situational levels, we can also view goals at two levels: superordinate or situational (Stein, Trabasso, & Liwag, 1992, 1994). Superordinate goals are overarching goals that are formed from our deepest sense of who we are. They provide the framework for situational goals. Superordinate goals are not always explicitly defined; they are often implicit and revealed through the sum of actions taken across situations. The following statement summarizes one caregiver's overarching, superordinate goal: "I try to be with him and hold his hand, kiss his forehead, rub his feet and let him know he is safe. I want to do that for him. I've made that commitment. I know he'd do that for me."

Situational goals are linked to the events of everyday life. They are derived from and in the service of superordinate goals. One caregiver said, "I have to deal with his mental and physical state and be careful about how often I go out, making sure someone is around so he won't wander or fall down." Situational goals also inform us as to whether we are acting consistently with our fundamental beliefs, values, and goals. Success or failure of situational goals, and our emotional response to the success or failure, provides feedback for interpreting how we are doing vis à vis our fundamental meaning structure. Based on our reflections, we reinstate or revise our beliefs about the situation and, more globally, our beliefs about our selves.

Two Case Studies

We argue that response shift is a process that depends in part on the individual's ability to recognize that previously valued expectations are no longer tenable, relinquish those expectations, and substitute new ones that are meaningful. We have selected two cases to illustrate these processes in significant real-life situations and the consequences of these processes with respect to response shift.

For each participant in our study there was a point at which treatment was no longer effective or tolerable, and the ill partner began moving toward death. The decision as to when the terminal stage began was made either by the physician, the patient, or the caregiving partner, or it was made collaboratively. For both the patient and the caregiver, this determination provoked a sense of loss and sadness and, frequently, the awareness that some changes were necessary to accommodate this transition. The goal of fighting the disease was no longer available, and the focus shifted to comfort care and life closure issues.

When asked to recount what occurred at the time of death, participants often began their narrative accounts with an event that they marked as the beginning of the end. The timing of this marker event ranged from within hours of the death to events that took place as much as one and a half years prior to the death. Theoretically, the awareness and engagement with life closure should lead to shifts in global and situational meaning, beliefs about the self and the partner, and the definition of goals. The following case studies of one participant who was aware of the process of dying and another participant who was not illustrate how awareness can lead to shifts in meaning, beliefs, and goals and facilitate response shift. The names used in the studies are pseudonyms.

Case Study 1

Jeff's partner had been placed in hospice care. The selection of hospice care signals the recognition that the patient is terminal, and curative treatments cease. We do not learn who was involved in the decision-making process to move the ill partner into palliative care, but we do see that the decision was made and accepted by both partners. Jeff's opening narrative reflects his primary goal in the situation: keeping his partner out of pain. It also reveals a more global belief, voiced with driving emotion, that he is the dying partner's advocate. His actions are consistent with his personal sense of self-responsibility. He believes his partner to be in pain and will do whatever is necessary.

> Paul's pain was getting more intense and I talked to the daytime hospice nurse and said, "Is there something we can do?" Then I called Dr. X and he seemed to be tap dancing around and saying, "Well, we have in mind Xanax." And a psychiatrist had seen Paul and had him on some other drug and said, "You shouldn't put him on Xanax because the two might be in conflict." I thought, who cares if there's a conflict, as long as he's not in pain. I mean the man's dying! Who cares if he leaves town with a drug habit?

Jeff's awareness of Paul's pending death moved him toward a closer attunement to his partner:

> I was talking with friends and all of a sudden I just got this strange feeling that I needed to go see Paul. So I jumped in the truck and I said, "I'll see you guys later," and drove over and parked the truck and walked in. And I said, "Sweetie, I'm here," and he went (imitates gasp), and that was it. That was the last breath.

Jeff's awareness and acceptance of Paul's impending death also influenced the dyadic relationship, allowing closure to take place over some period of time prior to the death. In their own humorous way, Jeff and Paul were also able to speak of their spiritual beliefs of an afterlife.

> I went and I sat down with Paul and picked his hand up and told him how much I loved him and that I would miss him. And the thing that was good is that we really didn't have anything to say to one another. We had said it all. There were no feelings that I hadn't expressed. We used to joke about the fact that this was not the game plan. I was

> supposed to go first because I am older. I said, "Now it's your job to get to whatever the next level is and you find the house and get it furnished so that when I arrive, the strawberries and the champagne are ready and I don't have to go through any of the moving or putting stuff away." So it was good.

Through these processes, Jeff was able to relinquish his expectations that Paul would live and substitute new expectations and concordant goals regarding the nature of the time left to them. Jeff was thus able to sustain positive meaning. Given the deteriorating circumstances and Jeff's success at revising his beliefs, expectations, and goals, we take this as evidence of a response shift.

Case Study 2

Although Robert's partner was very ill, Robert did not believe that he would die soon. Because of this belief, which was at odds with reality, it was difficult for Robert to interpret events accurately. Robert's primary goals in the situation, based on his beliefs, were to get the necessary treatment for his partner and to bring his partner home. Robert's actions were consistent with his beliefs and goals in that he felt the freedom to leave the hospital in order to get some sleep and go to work the following day.

> Right before Christmas he went into the hospital and they gave him a blood transfusion and sent him home. Of course, we had to go to the emergency room and it was very traumatic, then they released him the next day. So then he came home and he didn't really get any better, he got worse. Tuesday he went back in the hospital and they diagnosed him as having pneumocystis again. I was really totally unprepared for his death I think. He had a really rough day and then they moved him to another unit and he had actually passed out. It was really breaking me up to see him doing so badly and I was really angry at the hospital. I'd seen him from 5:00 to 7:00 that night and he was breathing really heavily, having a hard time breathing. I went home to go to bed because I had to go to work and I did not think he was going to die. The following Thursday morning they called and said he's taken a turn for the worse, he'd had cardiac arrest. I flipped out and started crying. I got kind of hysterical. Then the grief just came over. It was like howling, wailing. I've never heard sounds come out of me like that. I was not prepared. There was nothing I could do. I was so angry that I had gone home, that I didn't see the signs.

When his partner died, Robert was completely overwhelmed, despite the numerous indicators that preceded the death. Robert's belief that there was nothing he could do in the situation meant he could not adopt an advocacy position that would allow him to open the necessary dialogue with medical staff to prepare for his partner's death. His belief also diminished the possibility of his achieving attunement with his partner. Robert emerged from the circumstance with enormous anger directed primarily at himself. He had failed to revise his beliefs and expectations in accordance with changing reality. As a consequence, he was unable to derive meaning from what had happened, which also meant that he lost the opportunity for maintaining any sense of well-being or finding solace to ease his initial grief reaction.

The circumstances of bereavement and the meanings attached to them are unique to each individual. There is typically a period of cognitive and emotional assimilation of the facts of death whereby those bereaved organize the events of death into a coherent story with acceptable meanings (Bowlby, 1980; Parkes & Weiss, 1983; Weiss, 1988). This is one part of the grieving process that helps people make sense of the events. In our studies on spirituality and loss (Richards, Acree, & Folkman, 1999; Richards & Folkman, 1997; Richards, Wrubel, & Folkman, 1999), we have found that spiritual beliefs and practices contribute to both coping and the meaning reconstruction process involved in grief.

In looking at the two case studies of bereavement, we see emotions, beliefs, goals, and actions that were bound in the interpretation and meaning of events as they occurred, affecting the response to the circumstances at hand. We also see how the mechanisms of response shift—the physical, psychological, social, and, in the first case, spiritual domains—can interact to produce very different responses from those of the participants in these studies. As these two individuals moved into the process of assimilation, they were faced with very different content to sort and interpret as they went about making sense of the facts of death. Within weeks of the loss, Jeff was able to say, "It was good." However, Robert was left with, "I was so angry that I had gone home, that I didn't see the signs." Although both men experienced loss and grief, one was also able to voice positive emotion and meaning concurrently.

Response Shift and Coping Theory

The concept of response shift is compatible with a recent revision of coping theory (Folkman, 1997). We describe the model here because we believe that it helps formalize the point we have made in our discussion and through the case histories about response shift and the processes through which it is achieved and sustained. The revised model is shown in Figure 2.1.

The model revolves around two processes—appraisal and coping—that are at the heart of the original stress and coping model (Lazarus & Folkman, 1984) that this revised model is based on. Appraisal refers to the individual's evaluation of the personal significance of a given event and the adequacy of his or her resources for coping. It influences emotion and subsequent coping. Coping refers to the thoughts and behaviors that a person uses to regulate distress (emotion-focused coping), to manage the problem causing distress (problem-focused coping), and to maintain positive well-being (meaning-based coping). Coping influences the outcome of the situation and the individual's appraisal of it.

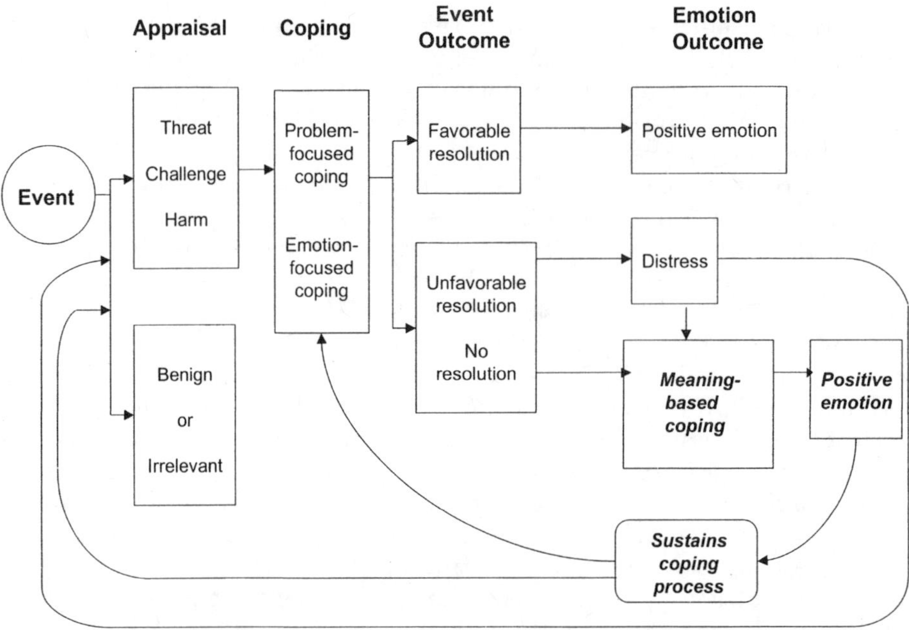

Figure 2.1. A revised model of coping theory. Reprinted from "Positive Psychological States and Coping With Severe Stress," by S. Folkman, 1997, *Social Science and Medicine, 45*(8), pp. 1207–1221. Copyright 1997 by Elsevier Science. Reprinted with permission.

The appraisal process is based on the assumption that people are constantly evaluating their relationship to the environment, and the stress process begins when the person becomes aware of a change or a threatened change in the status of current goals and concerns. The appraisal includes an evaluation of the personal significance of the change, which is called "primary appraisal," and an evaluation of the options for coping, which is called "secondary appraisal." The appraisal process influences subsequent coping. Greater control (secondary appraisal) is associated with higher levels of problem-focused coping, such as information seeking, problem solving, and taking direct action to solve a problem. Less control is associated with higher levels of emotion-focused coping, such as escape and avoidance, seeking social support, distancing, or cognitive reframing.

Events that are brought to a clear conclusion lead to an appraisal of the outcome as being favorable or unfavorable. A favorable event outcome is likely to lead to a benefit appraisal, positive emotion, and the conclusion of coping activity. An unsatisfactory outcome (e.g., an unfavorable resolution or no resolution), as in the case of a chronic and unremittingly stressful condition, is likely to lead to a stress appraisal of harm, loss, or threat (most likely in combination), distress emotion, and the need for additional coping. Distress, even the most intense distress, sets the stage for meaning-based coping processes that generate positive affect, thereby providing relief from distress.

In the Sprangers and Schwartz model (see chapter 1), coping is one mechanism contributing to response shift. We believe that when response shift occurs, it is as a result of specific meaning-based coping processes that come into play when previous beliefs, expectations, and goals are no longer tenable. The coping processes that we posit are necessary for response shift involve the realistic appraisal of changing circumstances, the consequent need to revise beliefs and expectations at both global and situational levels, and the adoption of new expectations and goals that are realistic and meaningful at both global and situational levels. To achieve a stable response shift, this process probably needs to be enacted repeatedly over specific stressful situations related to the ongoing chronic condition. This conceptualization is consistent with Sprangers and Schwartz's model of coping as one of the mechanisms that supports response shift.

Conclusion

In this chapter, we provided a framework for thinking about the mechanisms of response shift. At the center of our discussion was the importance of making meaning in the face of adversity. This is not a new idea, but it is an important one to be reminded of, especially in the context of recent psychology that has been so much concerned with the distress that life's difficulties bring. In describing his experiences in concentration camps, Viktor Frankl (1959, p. 64) called the phenomenon of meaning making "practicing the art of living." Practicing the art of living involves finding personal meaning and still beholding the goodness in life, even when circumstances become horrific and seemingly unrelenting. Frankl believed that, as human beings, we cannot directly grasp the greater Meaning of our lives. However, he felt that if we engaged in the smaller meanings in life and experienced the joys of those meanings, we might catch an oblique glance at Meaning. In these ideas, Frankl expressed the essential elements of emotional survival under adverse circumstances.

References

Andrykowski, M. A., Brady, M. J., & Hunt, J. W. (1993). Positive psychosocial adjustment in potential bone marrow transplant recipients: Cancer as a psychosocial transition. *Psycho-Oncology, 2,* 261–276.

Antonovsky, A. (1987). *Unraveling the mystery of health.* San Francisco: Jossey-Bass.

Baumeister, R. F. (1991). *Meanings of life.* New York: Guilford Press.

Bowlby, J. (1980). *Attachment and loss: Loss, sadness and depression* (Vol. 3). New York: Basic Books.

Breetvelt, I. S., & van Dam, F. S. A. M. (1991). Underreporting by cancer patients: The case of response shift. *Social Science and Medicine, 32,* 981–987.

Carver, C. S., & Scheier, M. F. (1998). *On the self-regulation of behavior.* New York: Cambridge University Press.

Csikszentmihalyi, M. (1990). *Flow: The psychology of optimal experience.* New York: Harper & Row.

Emmons, R. A., & Kaiser, H. A. (1996). Goal orientation and emotional well-being: Linking goals and affect through the self. In L. L. Martin & A. Tesser (Eds.), *Striving and feeling* (pp. 79–98). Mahwah, NJ: Erlbaum.

Folkman, S. (1997). Positive psychological states and coping with severe stress. *Social Science and Medicine, 45*(8), 1207–1221.

Folkman, S., Chesney, M. A., & Christopher-Richards, T. A. (1994). Stress and coping in caregiving partners of men with AIDS. *Psychiatric Clinics of North America, 17,* 35–53.

Folkman, S., Chesney, M. A., Collette, L., Boccellari, A., & Cooke, M. (1996). Post-bereavement depressive mood and its pre-bereavement predictors in HIV+ and HIV- gay men. *Journal of Personality and Social Psychology, 70,* 336–348.

Folkman, S., Moskowitz, J., Ozer, E., & Park, C. (1997). Positive meaningful events and coping in the context of HIV/AIDS. In B. Gottlieb (Ed.), *Coping with chronic stress* (pp. 293–314). New York: Plenum Press.

Folkman, S., & Stein, N. L. (1996). A goal-process approach to analyzing narrative memories for AIDS-related stressful events. In N. Stein, P. Ornstein, B. Tversky, & C. Brainerd (Eds.), *Memory for everyday and emotional events* (pp. 113–137). Hillsdale, NJ: Erlbaum.

Frankl, V. (1959). *Man's search for meaning.* New York: Washington Square Press.

Lazarus, R. S., & Folkman, S. (1984). *Stress, appraisal, and coping.* New York: Springer.

Park, C. L., & Folkman, S. (1997). Meaning in the context of stress and coping. *Review of General Psychology, 1*(2), 115–144.

Parkes, C. M., & Weiss, R. (1983). *Recovery from bereavement.* New York: Basic Books.

Reker, G. T., & Wong, P. T. (1988). Aging as an individual process: Toward a theory of personal meaning. In J. E. Birren & V. L. Bengston (Eds.), *Emerging theories of aging* (pp. 214–246). New York: Springer.

Richards, T. A., Acree, M., & Folkman, S. (1999). Spiritual aspects of loss among partners of men with AIDS: Postbereavement follow-up. *Death Studies, 23*(2), 105–127.

Richards, T. A., & Folkman, S. (1997). Spiritual aspects of loss at the time of a partner's death from AIDS. *Death Studies, 21,* 527–552.

Richards, T. A., Wrubel, J., & Folkman, S. (1999). Death rites in the San Francisco gay community: Cultural developments of the AIDS epidemic. *Omega, Journal of Death and Dying, 40*(2), 313–329.

Stein, N. L., Folkman, S., Trabasso, T., & Richards. T. A. (1997). Appraisal and goal processes as predictors of well-being in bereaved caregivers. *Journal of Personality and Social Psychology, 72,* 872–884.

Stein, N. L., Trabasso, T., & Liwag, M. (1992). The representation and organization of emotional experience. Unfolding the emotional episode. In M. Lewis & J. Haviland (Eds.), *Handbook of emotion* (pp. 279–299). New York: Guilford Press.

Stein, N. L., Trabasso, T., & Liwag, M. (1994). The Rashomon phenomenon: Personal frames and future-oriented appraisals in memory for emotional events. In M. Haith (Ed.), *Future-oriented processes* (pp. 409–435). Chicago: University of Chicago Press.

Weiss, R. (1988). Loss and recovery. *Journal of Social Issues, 44,* 37–52.

3

Response Shifts in Prostate Cancer Patients: An Evaluation of Suppressor and Buffer Models

Stephen J. Lepore and David T. Eton

Prostate Cancer as a Model for Studying Response Shifts and Quality of Life

Individuals afflicted with life-threatening or disabling illness report a very positive or stable quality of life (QOL) with surprisingly high frequency. Schwartz and Sprangers (see chapters 1 and 6) have invoked the concept of response shifts to help explain such paradoxical findings. They define response shifts as a change in the meaning of one's self-evaluation of QOL as a result of a change in one's internal standards of measurement (i.e., recalibration), the importance attributed to component domains constituting QOL (i.e., change in values), or construal of the meaning of QOL (i.e., concept redefinition). As a result of these shifts, individuals can appear to sustain a very high subjective QOL despite negative changes in their physical health.[1]

In this chapter, we examine response shifts as they relate to QOL in patients with prostate cancer. Cancer patients, including those with chronic treatment-related illness and dysfunction, often report that their QOL is equal to or superior to that of individuals without cancer or with

---

Work on this chapter was supported by National Institute of Health Grant CA68354 awarded to Stephen J. Lepore and National Institute of Mental Health Grant T32 MH19953 awarded to David T. Eton.

We acknowledge the important contributions of co-investigators Jeffrey Cohen, Thomas Hakala, Vicki Helgeson, Ronald Hrebinko, Raoul Salup, and Richard Schulz. We thank our research staff—Michelle Bruno, Michael Mattis, Renee Rhodes, and Timothy Roberts—as well as our consultants—Ronald Benoit, Leslie Bonci, Adam Brufsky, Stephen Campanella, John Franz, Scott Long, Jay Lutins, Ralph Miller, Lynn Roberts, Robert Schwartz, and Donald Trump. We are grateful to Carolyn Schwartz for introducing us to the concept of response shift, helping us see its relevance to our work, and giving us invaluable feedback on this chapter. We also thank Bruce Rapkin and Mirjam Sprangers for their insightful comments on an earlier draft of this chapter.

[1]Response shifts could result in negative changes in self-evaluations of QOL. Our chapter focuses on explaining the potential positive influences of response shift on self-evaluations of QOL.

less severe illness (e.g., Andrykowski, Brady, & Hunt, 1993; Lepore, in press; Lepore & Helgeson, 1998a; Litwin et al., 1995). Perhaps response shifts can help explain why having cancer, or experiencing severe and negative side effects from cancer, does not appear to undermine QOL in many patients (see Breetvelt & van Dam, 1991). We propose that response shifts reflect cognitive processes that enhance or sustain QOL in people facing serious health problems, such as cancer.

Prostate cancer is the second leading cause of cancer death among American men (American Cancer Society, 1998). Many prostate tumors are indolent, but aggressive ones can result in death in months. Fortunately, modern technologies for detecting and controlling prostate cancer have spared many men from untimely deaths. However, even if cured of prostate cancer, patients can experience intense and enduring physical complications related to their treatment (Lepore & Helgeson, 1998a).

The most common complications associated with prostate cancer and its treatment are sexual and urinary dysfunction. Litwin et al. (1995) found that, compared to men without prostate cancer in an age-matched control group, men treated for prostate cancer reported significantly worse sexual and urinary function. Problems in sexual function included decreases in frequency of erections, quality of erections, and ability to achieve sexual climax. Urinary problems included greater frequency and amounts of leakage. Others (Adolfsson, Helgason, Dickman, & Steineck, 1998) have reported similar results. We would expect persistent problems in sexual and urinary functioning to have a profound negative effect on men's QOL. Yet the empirical data do not support this commonsensical notion. In addition to assessing physical complications associated with prostate cancer, Litwin et al. (1995) assessed men's QOL in many domains, including social relationships, physical and role functions, and emotional well-being. They found no differences in QOL between men with prostate cancer and their cancer-free counterparts. Other investigators have found that men treated for prostate cancer actually reported higher QOL than did similarly aged men without prostate cancer (Frazer, Brown, & Graves, 1998) or men with benign prostate problems (Lepore & Helgeson, 1998b).

Despite the physical complications associated with prostate cancer and its treatment, men with prostate cancer often do not report a worse QOL than similarly aged men without cancer, men with other prostate problems, or normal populations without cancer. This discontinuity between physical health and QOL is precisely the phenomenon that Schwartz and Sprangers have attempted to explain with the response shift construct. Therefore, prostate cancer provides a good model for examining the role of response shifts in QOL.

Suppressor and Buffering Models of Response Shifts and QOL

In this chapter, we investigate two hypothetical models of the role of response shifts in QOL among men recovering from prostate cancer treatments. We formulated these models based on the emerging theory of response shifts developed by Sprangers and Schwartz (see chapter 1 for a full discussion). According to one model, the suppressor model, response shifts can suppress the relation between physical health problems and QOL. According to the buffering model, response shifts can moderate, or buffer, the relation between physical health problems and QOL. These two models are illustrated in Figure 3.1 (for detailed discussions of suppressor and moderator models, see Baron & Kenny, 1986; Cohen & Cohen, 1983; Evans & Lepore, 1997). Both models can be used to explain how response shifts can attenuate the relation between physical health problems and QOL and how response shifts can be viewed as a potentially adaptive mechanism.

According to the suppressor model, physical health problems act as a catalyst to response shifts. That is, physical health problems stimulate response shifts by causing people to recalibrate their QOL, change their values, or change the meaning of QOL. Response shifts, in turn, sustain or enhance QOL. There are several assumptions of this model that can be tested statistically. First, response shifts should be strongest in people who experience the greatest negative changes in health. Second, response

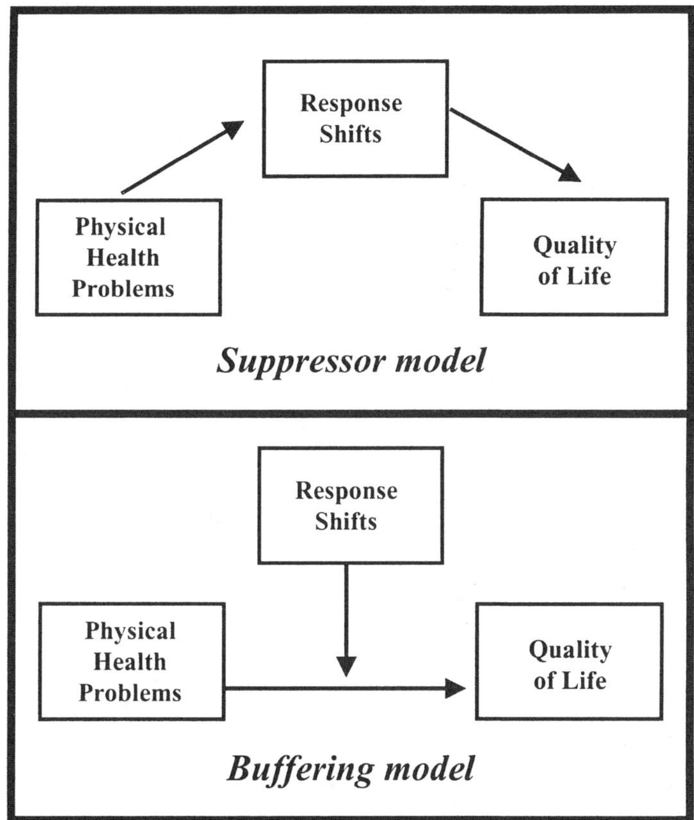

Figure 3.1. Schematic of the suppressor (top panel) and buffering (bottom panel) models of response shift.

shifts should be associated with positive QOL outcomes. Third, to the extent that response shifts suppress the association between health problems and QOL, we should observe a negative relation between health problems and QOL only when the effects of response shifts have been statistically controlled (i.e., using analysis of covariance techniques).

According to the buffering model, response shifts moderate (i.e., attenuate) the negative association between physical health problems and QOL (Schwartz et al., 1999; see also chapter 1). The buffering model assumes that response shifts can be stimulated by mechanisms such as coping styles and social support. From this perspective, some individuals with health problems will exhibit response shifts, and others will not. The model further assumes that health problems will be associated with a poorer QOL in individuals who do not make response shifts but not in individuals who do make response shifts. The primary criterion for testing this model statistically is evidence of an interactive effect of response shifts and health problems on QOL. Specifically, health problems should be associated with poorer QOL in individuals who do not make response shifts and unrelated to QOL in individuals who do make such shifts.

Note that the general theory of response shift being developed by Schwartz and Sprangers can accommodate both buffer and suppressor effects. In other words, these models are not mutually exclusive. It is possible that changes in health status can act as a catalyst to response shifts *and* interact with response shifts. For instance, individuals with more severe negative health changes might make more extreme response shifts than will individuals with relatively minor health changes. Yet, at the same time, response shifts may be critical in buffering the effects of health problems on QOL. Furthermore, it is possible that changes in health status and interpersonal (e.g., social support) or intrapersonal (e.g., coping style) mechanisms can stimulate response shifts.

In testing these models, we focused on two components of response shift: recalibration of internal standards for measuring QOL and changes in values. Because investigations into response shifts and QOL are relatively new, there is little known about which measures are most reliable or valid. Furthermore, it is not known whether different aspects of response shifts influence QOL in the same way. For these and other reasons, it is desirable to include more than one indicator of response shifts in QOL research (see chapter 6).

Recalibration of Internal Standards

Recalibration reflects a change in the individual's internalized standards for measuring QOL. According to the suppressor model, negative changes in health status may cause people to change their internal standards for measuring QOL (cf. Breetvelt & van Dam, 1991). In turn, this recalibration of internal standards can result in stable or higher QOL in individuals over time.

To illustrate this process, we can consider how recalibration might suppress the association between health problems and QOL in a prostate cancer patient. Prior to being diagnosed with prostate cancer, a patient might rate his anxiety as moderate. At the time of diagnosis, the patient might realize that his life is at risk and consequently rate his anxiety as high. After having his prostate removed, the patient may experience complications such as sexual dysfunction and incontinence but may rate his anxiety as only moderate relative to the high anxiety brought on by the diagnosis. Furthermore, in retrospect he might reevaluate his original anxiety as being low rather than moderate, because the anchors and intervals for evaluating anxiety have changed as a result of having a life-threatening diagnosis. Thus, the rating of moderate anxiety has different meanings to the patient at different points in time. Furthermore, as a result of the recalibration, the patient's rating of anxiety from prediagnosis to posttreatment looks stable, even though his physical functioning is objectively worse posttreatment.

In the buffering model, recalibration is conceived of as an individual difference variable, perhaps driven by interpersonal (e.g., social support) or intrapersonal (e.g., coping style) mechanisms. The model maintains that when recalibration occurs, it can attenuate the association between health problems and QOL. To illustrate these processes, we can consider how recalibration might attenuate the negative association between health problems and QOL in a patient with prostate cancer. In this illustration, we identify downward social comparisons (Wood & Van Der Zee, 1997) as a coping style that could influence QOL through scale recalibration.

A prostate cancer patient engaging in downward social comparisons might scan the social environment to identify patients in worse physical condition than his own. This process can lead him to expand his internal scale to account for worse outcomes. For example, a patient who initially perceives that his role functioning is poor might upgrade his self-evaluation of role functioning after identifying individuals with worse role functioning. These changes in evaluation of role functioning can occur even though the patient's objective role functioning has not changed. Furthermore, the patient could apply this positive reevaluation of role functioning to both his current state and his state prior to making social comparisons. In contrast, a patient who does not engage in downward social comparisons might not recalibrate his internal standards for evaluating QOL. Such a patient would not exhibit a positive change in his QOL.

Changes in Values

Similarly, we can speculate on how changes in values can act as a suppressor or buffer of the relation between health problems and QOL. A cancer diagnosis can evoke an existential crisis in some individuals. This may lead to a search for meaning in life (Silver, Boon, & Stones, 1983) and a reordering of life's priorities (Rapkin & Fischer, 1992). For others, the negative side effects and life threat associated with cancer might challenge fundamental life goals. As a result of reevaluating the feasibility and importance of achieving certain goals, cancer patients might reorder or change important life goals (for a detailed discussion of goal constructs and goal restructuring, see Austin & Vancouver, 1996). We believe that changes in primary goals are accompanied by changes in individuals' basic values in life. That is, changing primary goals involves a fundamental cognitive restructuring, or transformation, of basic beliefs about what is good and important in life.

Although cancer can undermine QOL by robbing people of meaning and threatening life goals, changing values can help people to restore meaning (i.e., by identifying something important in life) and defuse goal threats (i.e., by changing or reordering goals). In this way, changes in values might help patients to accommodate to limitations imposed by their illness. These processes could enhance QOL by changing the implications the illness has for their QOL (i.e., the precursors to QOL). Changes in values may influence the relation between health problems and QOL through suppressor or buffering effects. The Sprangers and Schwartz model of response shifts suggests that health problems can be a catalyst, or stimulus, for change in values. If changes in values occur as a normative response to health problems, then we would expect these changes to suppress the association between health problems and QOL. That is, health problems would trigger changes in values, which in turn would enhance QOL. On the other hand, if the tendency to change values is an individual difference variable, then we would expect to see interactive effects of changes in values and health problems on QOL. Specifically, health problems will be associated with poorer QOL outcomes among patients who do not make value changes than among patients who do make such changes.

A Study of Response Shifts Among Cancer Patients

We evaluated the suppressor and buffering models in men who had been treated for nonmetastatic prostate cancer. We investigated whether two aspects of response shifts—recalibration of internal standards and changes in values—act as suppressors or buffers of the association between cancer-related health problems and QOL. Following recommendations by Schwartz and Sprangers (see chapter 6), we assessed recalibration of internal standards using the thentest approach and assessed changes in values using a measure of primary life goal changes (see also chapters 4 and 9 for other examples using these methods). Physical health problems were assessed with a measure of urinary and sexual dysfunction, because these are the primary physical complications resulting from prostate cancer treatments. QOL was assessed with a standardized measure of social–emotional functioning.

Based on the suppressor model, we predicted that prostate cancer patients experiencing worsening health problems would be more likely to make response shifts than would men whose health improved (i.e., health problems are a catalyst of response shifts). We tested this hypothesis by examining whether changes in health problems (e.g., urinary and sexual dysfunction) were associated with recalibration of internal standards or changes in values. The suppressor model also asserts that response shifts mediate (suppress) the association between health problems and QOL. We tested this hypothesis by examining whether the associations between changes in health problems and changes in QOL increased after statistically controlling for the effects of response shift (i.e., covarying recalibration and changes in values).

Based on the buffering model, we predicted that prostate cancer patients experiencing worsening health problems (e.g., sexual or urinary dysfunction) and engaging in response shifts would report greater improvements in their QOL than would their counterparts who do not make response shifts. We tested this hypothesis by examining the interactive effects of response shift and changes in health status on changes in QOL.

Method

Participants and Procedure

Data were collected from 166 men who had been treated for nonmetastatic prostate cancer. All men were participating in a larger study on the effects of education and social support on QOL in men treated for prostate cancer. The results of the intervention study will be reported elsewhere, as they did not affect the findings reported herein. The mean age of the men was 65. The racial distribution was 86.7% White, 12.7% Black, and 0.6% Asian. Most (83.7%) of the men were married. Medical treatments for prostate cancer included radical prostatectomy (53.6%), brachytherapy (19.9%), pelvic irradiation (17.5%), cryosurgery (4.8%), or a combination of brachytherapy and pelvic irradiation (4.2%). We collected data on QOL, physical health problems, and response shifts in two structured, face-to-face interviews, spaced 10 weeks apart. The first interview took place approximately one month after the treatment start date and six months after diagnosis.

Measures

Quality of life: The mental component score of the SF-12. We used the 12-item version of the Medical Outcomes Study Short-Form General Health Survey (SF-12; Ware, Kosinski, & Keller, 1995) to assess perceived QOL at Time 1 (T1) and Time 2 (T2). The SF-12 provides an aggregate mental component summary (MCS) score, which reflects QOL in the social–emotional domain (i.e., social and emotional functioning, vitality, role functioning). Sample items include "During the past 4 weeks, how much of the time has your physical health or emotional problems interfered with your social activities?" "During the past 4 weeks, how often have you felt calm and peaceful?" and "During the past 4 weeks, have you accomplished less than you would have liked as a result of an emotional problem?" The measure has good psychometric properties and has been well-validated (Ware et al., 1995). Scores are standardized and range from a low of 0 to a high of 100, with a higher score indicative of better QOL.

Physical health problems: The Prostate Cancer Index. We used the UCLA Prostate Cancer Index (PCI; Litwin et al., 1998) to assess physical health problems (urinary and sexual dysfunction) at T1 and T2. A sample item from the urinary functioning scale is "Over the past 4 weeks, how often have you leaked urine?" A sample item from the sexual functioning scale is "How would you describe the quality of your erections in the last 4 weeks?" The two subscales have good psychometric properties and validity (Litwin et al., 1998). Scores range from 0 to 100, with higher scores indicative of more problems in urinary or sexual functioning.

Response shift: Recalibration. We used the thentest methodology to assess changes in internal standards of evaluating QOL (see chapter 6). Accordingly, men completed the SF-12 at T1 using conventional instructions. They also completed the SF-12 at T2 using the thentest instructions. Specifically, at T2 they were instructed to think back to the T1 interview period and answer the questions based on their QOL at that time (i.e., "then"). A response shift is indicated by a difference between men's original T1 and retrospective T1 reports of their QOL [thentest SF-12 score − T1 SF-12 score]. This difference can be either positive or negative. A positive difference indicates that, in retrospect (at T2), men reported their T1 QOL to be better than what they originally reported at T1. A negative difference indicates that in retrospect men reported their T1 QOL to be worse than what they originally reported at T1.

Response shift: Changes in values. We administered open-ended questions at T1 and T2 to assess whether men made changes in values. This was operationalized by looking at changes in primary life goals because such changes are likely to be reflective of a fundamental cognitive restructuring about what is good and important in life. Men were asked to report on their central life goal. The interviewer read the following instructions to determine men's central life goal: "I'd like you to take a second and think about the major goals in your life for the next year. What is the most important thing you would like to accomplish or achieve over the next year?" If more than one life goal was identified, men were asked to identify the single-most important goal. This procedure was modeled after one used by Rapkin (see Rapkin & Fischer, 1992; Rapkin et al., 1994).

Goals were summarized into a list from which we identified 11 global dimensions. Judges independently coded goals as belonging to one of these dimensions. Interrater reliability was good (kappa = .86). Examples of goal dimensions include leisure/hobbies (e.g., travel), self-actualization (e.g., increase faith), financial (e.g., invest), social/interpersonal (e.g., spend more time with family), and health goals (e.g., stay healthy).

Data Analytic Approach

We used a combination of correlation and regression analyses to test the suppressor and buffering models. Because we were interested in predicting changes in QOL based on changes in health status and response shifts, we first computed some change scores. We computed a QOL change score using the T1 and T2 SF-12 scores (T2 SF-12 score − T1 SF-12 score). Higher scores on the QOL difference index reflect improvements in QOL from T1 to T2. We then created four predictor variables. Two of the predictors were indicators of response shifts. We computed recalibration using the thentest and T1 SF-12 scores (thentest SF-12 score − T1 SF-12 score). Higher scores on this measure mean that men's retrospective (i.e., "then") reports of their QOL were more positive than their original (T1) reports. Lower scores indicate that men's retrospective reports of their QOL were more negative than their original reports. We created a dichotomous index of change in values by coding whether life goals changed over time (0 = same primary life goal at T1 and T2; 1 = different primary life goal at T1 and T2). The other two predictors were indicators of changes in health status based on the PCI: changes in urinary function (T1 urinary functioning − T2 urinary functioning) and changes in sexual function (T1 sexual functioning − T2 sexual functioning). Higher scores indicate that men reported improvements in sexual and urinary functioning over time.

The main goal of the suppressor analyses is to test whether a null relation between negative health status changes and QOL can be explained by response shifts. This can be demonstrated statistically in two steps: (1) show that negative changes in urinary and sexual functioning are unrelated to changes in QOL over time when the response shift variables are left free to vary, and (2) show that negative changes in urinary and sexual functioning are associated with negative changes in QOL after the effects of response shifts are statistically controlled. We used regression analyses to test these relations. We repeated the analyses for each health problem indicator (i.e., changes in urinary problems, changes in sexual problems) and for each response shift indicator (i.e., recalibration, changes in goals). For instance, we regressed changes in QOL on changes in urinary functioning with and without recalibration entered as a covariate. We used correlation analyses to test the viability of other assumptions of the suppressor model, including the assumption that negative changes in urinary and sexual functioning would act as a catalyst of response shifts and that response shifts would be associated with better QOL.

We used a series of moderated regression analyses (Aiken & West, 1991; Lunnenborg, 1994) to test the predictions of the buffering model. The aim of these analyses was to determine whether the relation between changes in sexual or urinary problems and changes in QOL was weaker among men who make response shifts than among men who do not make response shifts. We computed separate regression analyses for each health problem indicator (i.e., changes in urinary problems, changes in sexual problems). We used separate regression analyses to evaluate the moderating role of recalibration and changes in values, respectively. For instance, we regressed changes in QOL on changes in urinary functioning, changes in life goals, and the cross product of changes in urinary functioning × changes in life goals. Significant interactions were plotted to interpret whether the effects were consistent with buffering.

Results

The regression analyses did not support the suppressor model. Change in QOL was unrelated to increases in urinary and sexual problems either with or without the response shift variables entered as covariates. Furthermore, increases in urinary and sexual functioning were not correlated with response shifts when operationalized as changes in life goals and recalibration of QOL (see Table 3.1). There was a positive relation between QOL recalibration and change in QOL over time, but life goal change was not significantly related to change in QOL.

Next, we tested the buffering model. First, we tested whether changes in life goals attenuate the relation between negative changes in physical functioning (i.e., urinary and sexual functioning) and QOL. We found a significant urinary function change × life goal change interaction (beta = −.14, p < .05). As is shown in Figure 3.2, men whose urinary functioning worsened over time had improved QOL if they changed their life goal and decrements in QOL if they did not change their goal. Changes in sexual functioning did not interact with changes in life goals.

Second, we tested whether scale recalibration attenuates the relation between negative changes in physical functioning (urinary and sexual functioning) and QOL. We found a main effect of recalibration on QOL (beta = .65, $p < .001$). Specifically, men who made a large positive recalibration of their T1 QOL reported larger increases in their QOL by T2 than did men who made a relatively small positive recalibration of their T1 QOL. Men who made a large negative recalibration of their T1 QOL reported larger decreases in their QOL by T2 than men who made a relatively small negative recalibration of their T1 QOL. This main effect was qualified by a marginally significant urinary function change × recalibration interaction (beta = −.12, $p < .06$). As is shown in Figure 3.3, men whose urinary functioning worsened over time had decrements in QOL if

Table 3.1. Intercorrelations of Functioning, Response Shift, and Quality of Life (QOL) in Six Prostate Cancer Patients

Variable	1	2	3	4	5
1. Urinary function change	—	.09	.04	.08	.14
2. Sexual function change		—	.23**	−.04	.12
3. Life goal change			—	.20*	.15
4. Recalibration of QOL				—	.63**
5. QOL change					—

Note. *$p < .05$, two-tailed. **$p < .01$, two-tailed.

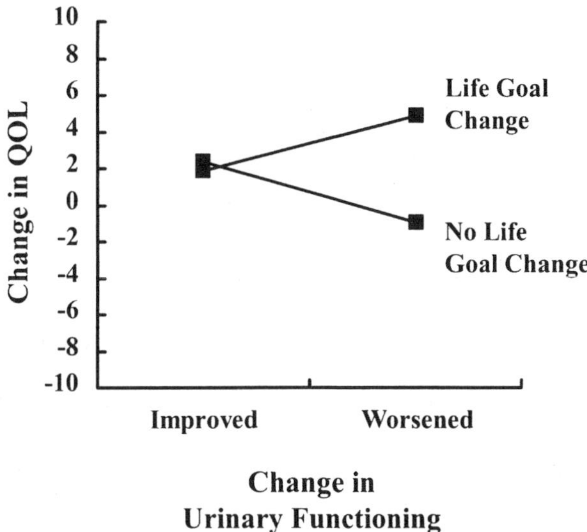

Figure 3.2. Slopes of the relation between changes in urinary function (T1 − T2) and changes in QOL (T2 SF-12 − T1 SF-12) among prostate cancer patients as a function of change in primary life goals (T1 − T2).

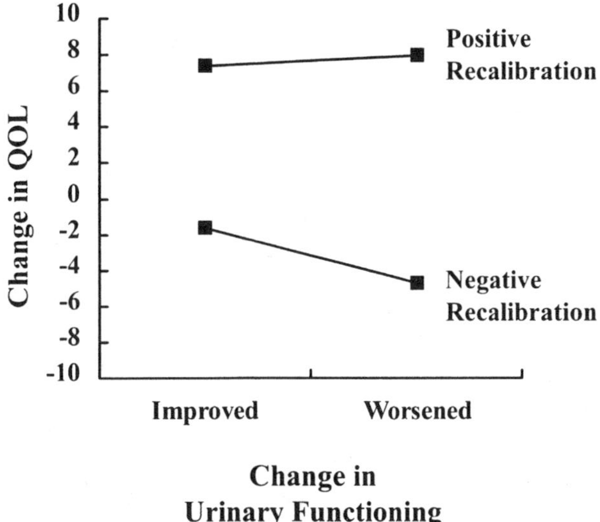

Figure 3.3. Slopes of the relation between changes in urinary function (T1 − T2) and changes in QOL (T2 SF-12 − T1 SF-12) among prostate cancer patients as a function of recalibration of QOL (thentest SF-12 − T1 SF-12). Note: Positive scale recalibration is based on a recalibration score of +1 SD above the mean. A negative scale recalibration is based on a recalibration score of −1 SD below the mean.

they made a negative recalibration, but not if they made a positive recalibration. Changes in sexual functioning did not interact with recalibration.

Discussion

In this chapter, we identified two conceptual models of response shifts—the suppressor and buffer models—that could account for the frequently observed lack of association between health problems and QOL in cancer patients. We tested these models in men who had been treated for localized prostate cancer, because prior research suggests that QOL is often stable and positive in these men, despite frequent problems with sexual and urinary functioning. Our analyses produced some evidence consistent with the buffering model. There was an interactive effect suggesting that response shifts moderated the association between increases in urinary functioning problems and changes in QOL. Specifically, response shifts appeared to buffer men from the negative effects of declines in urinary functioning and QOL over time. We found no evidence to support the suppressor model of response shifts. Overall, the results suggest that the response shift construct is valuable for accounting for individual differences in QOL among patients with prostate cancer who experience health complications after treatment.

The null results from the suppressor model analyses can be interpreted in several ways. First, it is possible that health problems do not act as a catalyst of response shifts. We found that neither urinary nor sexual complications were associated with response shifts (i.e., recalibration, changes in values). We can tentatively conclude that health problems may be a necessary condition for response shifts (i.e., all people who make response shifts have health problems), but not a sufficient condition (i.e., not all people who have health problems make response shifts). This raises an interesting question about what factors might trigger response shifts. In their theory of response shifts, Sprangers and Schwartz suggested a variety of potential triggers (e.g., coping style, social support, and social comparison).

Second, it is possible that the timing of our measurement prevented us from observing an association between health problems and QOL. All measurement occurred in the first four months after men's treatment. If men perceived that the negative side effects of treatment were "normal" during this period, they might not have been inclined to make response shifts. That is, there would be no need to accommodate short-term complications. In addition, some men might have made response shifts before their treatment (i.e., after their diagnosis), rather than during the period under investigation. Our analyses would have coded these men as not making response shifts (i.e., no recalibration, no change in values).

A third explanation of the null results is that some men might not have perceived the side effects of incontinence or sexual dysfunction as a major problem. Men in this age cohort could have been dealing with urinary and sexual problems prior to their prostate cancer because of other physical or psychological conditions. To the extent that such men have already accommodated to these problems prior to their prostate cancer, they would have no need to make further accommodations after their treatment. In addition, some men might have perceived that urinary and sexual problems are a small price to pay if their cancer was cured.

There was reasonable evidence of buffering effects. Collectively, the findings of our moderated regressions support the conclusion that response shifts may sustain QOL in prostate cancer patients whose urinary functioning deteriorates. More generally, these findings suggest that response shifts may be cognitive accommodations to health problems, which help buffer individuals from the negative social–emotional consequences of health problems. Thus, when illness challenges particular values by thwarting relevant goals, individuals can adopt values and goals that are more attainable in their postmorbid state. Alternatively, individuals can alter the way they appraise their QOL, both in the present and the past, to enhance their QOL.

Our results also have practical implications for men recovering from prostate cancer treatments. We found that the negative influence of deteriorating urinary function on QOL could be buffered by changing important life goals, which we interpret to be a shift in values. Men who find controlling urinary function to be especially challenging may find that changing life goals helps them restore a sense of personal control in their lives. For example, a man who is preoccupied by the thought of leaking urine, or finds he must be cognizant of the location of the closest restroom facilities, may believe that his pursuit of career or work-related goals is less achievable (perhaps even less meaningful) than it was prior to treatment. By altering his principal goal in life to, for instance, spending more time with his wife, this man may be able to regain a sense of control over his life. The goal of relationship enhancement may seem more tangible and personally achievable despite problems with controlling urinary function. This change may help restore a patient's sense of control, meaning, and purpose in life, and hence serve as a means of accommodating to declines in physical functioning.

Furthermore, a recalibration of QOL may assist the cancer patient who is attempting to come to terms with worsening physical conditions. We found that among men whose urinary function worsened over time, a positive recalibration of QOL was associated with improvements in QOL, whereas a negative recalibration was associated with declines in QOL. Why should a positive recalibration of QOL be helpful? It is possible that such reappraisals of a previous state represent an adaptive cognitive bias. This bias can be considered adaptive because it functions to preserve a sense of emotional well-being even in the face of physical problems that may severely restrict activities. Such positive biases are commonly observed in both diseased and normal populations and appear to be somewhat protective of mental health (Taylor, 1989).

It is also possible, however, that memory itself may be biased. Specifically, memory for past appraisals of QOL may in some sense be biased by current appraisals. That is, memory for judgments of QOL in the past may be informed and perhaps even actively reconstructed using current evaluations of QOL (Levine, 1997). In this manner, positive evaluations of the present may provide a framework that encourages the overestimation of positive aspects of the past. Consequently, a patient's view of past QOL may be colored by current perception. Those who currently rate their QOL as being high may look at the past as being comparatively better than what they previously thought it was. Conversely, negative evaluations of the present might activate a negative evaluatory schema that encourages the overestimation of negative aspects of the past. Thus, a patient who currently rates QOL as low would be more likely to reassess the past as being comparatively worse than how it was previously perceived. In our sample of men treated for prostate cancer, we found some evidence for this explanation. Mean MCS scores at T2 were higher for men who positively reappraised T1 QOL (M = 55.6) versus those who negatively reappraised T1 QOL (M = 49.1).

In summary, we tested two models of response shift effects on QOL in men treated for prostate cancer. We did not find empirical evidence for the hypothesis that response shifts suppress the relation between changes in physical health problems and changes in QOL. We did find some evidence that response shifts moderate (i.e., buffer) the relation between health problems and QOL in men treated for prostate cancer. Specifically, the two aspects of response shift, scale recalibration and changes in values were found to moderate the relation between negative changes in physical health (i.e., increases in urinary functioning problems) and changes in QOL. Thus, response shifts may readily be identified as processes by which cancer patients accommodate to disease-induced deterioration in their physical function in order to preserve social and emotional well-being.

References

Adolfsson, J., Helgason, A. R., Dickman, P., & Steineck, G. (1998). Urinary and bowel symptoms in men with and without prostate cancer: Results from an observational study in the Stockholm area. *European Urology, 33,* 11–16.

Aiken, L. S., & West, S. G. (1991). *Multiple regression: Testing and interpreting interactions.* Newbury Park, CA: Sage.

American Cancer Society. (1998, December). *Prostate Cancer Resource Center* [On-line]. Available: www.cancer.org.

Andrykowski, M. A., Brady, M. J., & Hunt, J. W. (1993). Positive psychosocial adjustment in potential bone marrow transplant recipients: Cancer as a psychosocial transition. *Psycho-Oncology, 2,* 261–276.

Austin, J. T., & Vancouver, J. B. (1996). Goal constructs in psychology: Structure, process, and content. *Psychological Bulletin, 120,* 338–375.

Baron, R., & Kenny, D. A. (1986). The moderator–mediator variable distinction in social psychological research: Conceptual, strategic, and statistical considerations. *Journal of Personality and Social Psychology, 51,* 1173–1182.

Breetvelt, I. S., & van Dam, F. S. A. M. (1991). Underreporting by cancer patients: The case of response-shift. *Social Science & Medicine, 32,* 981–987.

Cohen, J., & Cohen, P. (1983). *Applied multiple regression/correlation analysis for the behavioral sciences* (2nd ed.). Hillsdale, NJ: Erlbaum.

Evans, G. W., & Lepore, S. J. (1997). Moderating and mediating processes in environment–behavior research. In G. T. Moore & R. W. Marans (Eds.), *Advances in environment, behavior, and design* (Vol. 4, pp. 255–285). New York: Plenum Press.

Frazer, G. H., Brown, C. H., & Graves, T. K. (1998). Assessment of QOL indicators among selected patients in a community cancer center. *Issues in Mental Health Nursing, 19,* 241–262.

Lepore, S. J. (in press). A social–cognitive processing model of emotional adjustment to cancer. In A. Baum & B. Andersen (Eds.), *Psychosocial interventions for cancer*. Washington, DC: American Psychological Association.

Lepore, S. J., & Helgeson, V. S. (1998a). Psychoeducational support group enhances QOL after prostate cancer. *Cancer Research, Therapy and Control, 28,* 1–11.

Lepore, S. J., & Helgeson, V.S. (1998b). Social constraints, intrusive thoughts, and mental health after prostate cancer. *Journal of Social & Clinical Psychology, 17,* 89–106.

Levine, L. J. (1997). Reconstructing memory for emotions. *Journal of Experimental Psychology: General, 126,* 165–177.

Litwin, M. S., Hays, R. D., Fink, A., Ganz, P. A., Leake, B., & Brook, R. H. (1998). The UCLA Prostate Cancer Index: Development, reliability, and validity of a health-related quality of life measure. *Medical Care, 36,* 1002–1012.

Litwin, M. S., Hays, R. D., Fink, A., Ganz, P. A., Leake, B., Leach, G. E., & Brook, R. H. (1995). Quality-of-life outcomes in men treated for localized prostate cancer. *Journal of the American Medical Association, 273,* 129–135.

Lunnenborg, C. E. (1994). *Modeling experimental and observational data*. Belmont, CA: Duxbury Press.

Rapkin, B. D., & Fischer, K. (1992). Personal goals of older adults: Issues in assessment and prediction. *Psychology & Aging, 7,* 127–137.

Rapkin, B. D., Smith, M. Y., Dumont, T., Correa, A., Palmer, S., & Cohen, S. (1994). Development of the idiographic functional status assessment: A measure of the personal goals and attainment activities of people with AIDS. *Psychology & Health, 9,* 111–129.

Schwartz, C. E., Foley, F. W., Rao, S. M., Bernardin, L. J., Lee, H., & Genderson, M. W. (1999). Stress and course of disease in multiple sclerosis. *Behavioral Medicine, 25*(3), 110–116.

Silver, R. L., Boon, C., & Stones, M. H. (1983). Searching for meaning in misfortune: Making sense of incest. *Journal of Social Issues, 39,* 81–102.

Taylor, S. E. (1989). *Positive illusions: Creative self-deception and the healthy mind.* New York: Basic Books.

Ware, J. E., Kosinski, M., & Keller, S. D. (1995). *SF-12: How to score the SF-12 physical and mental health summary scales* (2nd ed.). Boston: New England Medical Center, The Health Institute.

Wood, J. V., & Van Der Zee, K. (1997). Social comparisons among cancer patients: Under what conditions are comparisons upward and downward? In B. P. Buunk & F. X. Gibbons (Eds.), *Health, coping, and well-being: Perspectives from social comparison theory* (pp. 299–328). Mahwah, NJ: Erlbaum.

4

Personal Goals and Response Shifts: Understanding the Impact of Illness and Events on the Quality of Life of People Living With AIDS

Bruce D. Rapkin

Quality-of-life (QOL) assessment has come to play an increasingly important role in clinical decision making and treatment research. Despite a proliferation of work in instrument development, critical problems concerning definition, measurement, and interpretation of findings remain unresolved. Indeed, considerable experience with QOL instruments suggests that they may be insensitive and imprecise. For example, De Haes and van Knippenberg (1987) reviewed a number of studies in which cancer patients were compared to nonpatients and found few differences in subjective QOL measures. It is not uncommon for validated QOL measures to show weak or inconsistent treatment effects, to be insensitive to differences in morbidity, or to fail to converge with ratings made by family members or providers (Morris & Sherwood, 1987; Schipper, Clinch, McMurray, & Levitt, 1984).

In interpreting inconsistent findings such as these, it is generally assumed that QOL ratings greatly depend on a rater's frame of reference. This assumption begs several questions: What frames of reference do individuals use when asked to appraise their QOL? What factors influence different individuals' perspectives on QOL? How does an individual's frame of reference change over time? In this chapter I show how assessments of change in personal goals can be helpful for addressing these questions because they provide information about individuals' shifting frames of reference. Assessment of personal goals can help us appreciate more fully how illness and treatment affect QOL and explain some of the

This chapter is based on data from a larger study supported by an Agency for Health Care Policy and Research Grant awarded to Bruce Rapkin.

I thank Scott Cohen, Arlene Correa, Kimberly Dumont, Sarah Palmer, and Meredith Smith for their contributions to this study. I also thank Carolyn Schwartz and Mirjam Sprangers for their editorial assistance and consistent encouragement and support. They have led me to reconceptualize and recalibrate my standards for appraising editors and colleagues.

inconsistent findings common in the literature. I also explain how the impact of life events on QOL may be subject to response shifts associated with changes in personal goals, by drawing on the results of a longitudinal study of 140 people living with AIDS.

The Relation Between Personal Goals and QOL

Many authors over the past three decades have discussed the role that personal goals and related constructs play in the individual's conception of QOL. According to Cantril (1965), individuals evaluate their lives using subjective psychological criteria to anchor ratings of life satisfaction. These criteria may differ from person to person and from time to time. In their work on subjective well-being, Andrews and Withey (1976), George and Bearon (1980), and Diener (1984) have all described the appraisal of QOL as an evaluative process, involving a comparison between current circumstances and personal ideals. Campbell, Converse, and Rodgers (1976) noted the importance of establishing "absolute and interpersonally comparable measurement of aspiration" (p. 174) to understand the meaning of subjective well-being ratings. Calman (1984) defined QOL as "the difference, at a particular moment in time, between hopes and expectations and present experiences" (p. 125). Sartorius (1987) described QOL as the "anticipated satisfaction of personal goals" (p. 19). Cella and Tulsky (1990) have suggested that QOL refers to the "patients' appraisal of and satisfaction with their current level of functioning as compared to what they perceive to be possible or ideal" (p. 30). The common thread that binds these definitions is that self-reported QOL involves some subjective evaluation of goal attainment, the gap between what one has and what one wants in salient domains of life.

The goals that individuals use to define and anchor their subjective scales can change, thus causing a problem for QOL researchers. Studies usually hypothesize that treatments, disease progression, or life events have some consistent, linear impact on QOL evaluation. However, this sort of hypothesis ignores the implication of changing personal goals and concerns. For example, early in illness, an individual may want to return to perfect health and so may appraise global life satisfaction or subjective well-being against that standard. At a later point, the focus may be on pursuing sustainable levels of work and activities. Still later, the focus may be maintaining independent functioning at home. At each point, the individual has markedly different priorities and concerns in mind when evaluating QOL. Evaluative QOL scales provide no information about these changing priorities. Indeed, the individual may actually report the same level of QOL at each point in time. Such insensitivity to change in health status does not represent lack of validity or measurement error. Rather, ratings may be perfectly valid reflections of the individual's appraisal of the potential for goal attainment at the time they are made. It is the goals that have changed. Clearly, changes in goals may greatly complicate the ways in which health status is associated with change in QOL.

The Challenge of Assessing Goal Changes and Their Effects

To characterize how goals change over time, it is necessary to consider the problem of assessing goal content. The pervasive and far-reaching implications of health-related changes make it necessary to consider the goals related to every area of life. Research in the areas of personality and well-being has introduced a number of methods to delineate goal content, including both "ideographic" (Emmons, 1986; Klinger, Barta, & Maxleiner, 1980; Palys & Little, 1983) and "nomothetic" approaches (Bühler, Brind, & Horner, 1968). In this first study of the goals of people with AIDS, it made sense to begin with an ideographic approach that allowed respondents to describe goals and concerns in their own language. Indeed, it was necessary to conduct an open-ended assessment of goals as a prelude to developing a representative list of goals suitable to create a more standard, multi-item nomothetic assessment (Rapkin & Fischer, 1992). Ideographic assessment requires content analysis of verbatim responses to characterize the types of goals mentioned by each respondent. Shifts in goal content over time may be indicated by change in the number or importance of different types of goals.

Changes in health status and other life events may engender significant changes in an individual's personal goals. Such changes are intrinsically involved in the ways that individuals appraise their QOL and so can affect the apparent impact of events and health status changes on levels of QOL. Methods to assess personal goal content can be used to describe the goals that are most important to an individual and the ways those goals change from time to time. Thus, such changes can be taken into account in efforts to explain health-related QOL.

In terms of Sprangers and Schwartz's response shift model (see chapter 1), change in personal goals necessarily reflects two fundamental types of response shift: reconceptualization (e.g., different goals matter to me now) and reprioritization (e.g., the same goals matter, but they have changed in their relative importance). In regard to abstract, global aspects of QOL, such as satisfaction, general health, or emotional well-being, reconceptualization and reprioritization represent the shifting mix of concerns, challenges, and opportunities to cope that mark the illness trajectory. Among people with AIDS, who may have multiple social, psychological, and material unmet needs, emergent concerns and changing priorities may be dictated by more than the course of illness. It will be useful to consider how reconceptualization and reprioritization of key personal goals may be associated with change in QOL.

In general, a *response shift* in QOL may be operationally defined as a deviation of an observed score from some expected value, associated with a change in the way that individual appraises QOL. Regression models may be used to derive sample-specific expected values for QOL. For example, using multiple regression, it is possible to determine the impact of health status changes and other life events on QOL. The resulting regression equation provides an estimate of the expected QOL score for people in the sample, based on predictors in the model. Individuals who experience similar health status changes and stressful events are expected to change in their appraisals of QOL in exactly the same way. Residual variance caused by deviations from expected values is generally assumed to result from unspecified errors of measurement.

To detect response shift effects in this regression context, it is necessary to determine whether unexplained deviations, otherwise relegated to error, are associated with changes in personal goals. For example, remaining independent may become an increasingly important goal for some individuals. When health status declines, individuals who place a greater value on independence may experience more marked declines in QOL compared to others who do not share this goal. That difference in reaction, represented by deviations from expected QOL that can be explained by reprioritization or reconceptualization of goals, constitutes a response shift effect. In statistical terms, response shifts in QOL appear as significant interaction effects in a hierarchical regression analysis, when changes in goals moderate the impact of disease progression, life events, or treatments on QOL. Because interaction terms are entered following main effects in hierarchical regressions, this approach explicitly attempts to account for residual variance after expected QOL that is due to main effects for health status changes and after other events are taken into account.

Given the complex and dynamic relationship between personal goals and QOL, it is necessary to consider and rule out several competing ways that change in goals might be associated with residual change in QOL, prior to attributing variance to an event-by-goal interaction effect. First, it is possible that certain changes in goals are intrinsically adaptive (e.g., to increase positive activities) or maladaptive (e.g., to isolate oneself completely) in their own right and directly contribute to improved or diminished QOL. Thus, it is necessary to take main effects of goal changes into account. Second, a change in goals may lead individuals to mobilize or discard coping resources. Third, a change in goals may be associated with the initiation of personal efforts to cope. Each of these influences may be controlled statistically, before entering interaction terms into the regression models.

A Longitudinal Study of QOL Among People With AIDS

Participants and Procedures

To obtain a sample reflecting the mix of adult AIDS cases in New York City in 1993, we sampled patients from an outpatient virology clinic at a community hospital, a day treatment program primarily used by people with drug abuse histories and unstable housing, and an innovative inpatient treatment setting that involves patients' significant others in every aspect of care. Potential participants were informed about the purpose of the study and were offered $15 per interview as payment for their time. Interviews took approximately 60–90 minutes to complete, with breaks if necessary. If the patient agreed, we attempted to conduct the initial interview at the time of recruitment. Follow-up interviews were conducted at the original treatment setting or at a suitable location chosen by the patient (i.e., a restaurant, our office).

More than 90% of the patients approached for this study in the day treatment and virology clinic settings agreed to participate. Inpatients had a higher rate of nonparticipation (approximately 25%) because of acute illness and difficulty in scheduling the interview during their hospital stay. The original sample included 224 patients. Of these people, 84 were lost to follow-up, including 47 (56.0%) to death, 11 (13.1%) to illness, and 5 (5.6%) to refusal to continue. The remainder could not be contacted directly or through contacts they had provided. After six months, 140 (62.5% of the original sample; 79.1% of survivors) completed the follow-up interview.

My colleagues and I framed key questions about the role of personal goal assessment in health-related QOL research:

1. What are the personal goals of patients, and how do they change over time?
2. How are goal changes related to changes in health status and other life events?
3. Do changes in goals modify the impact of life events on QOL (indicating the presence of response shift effect)?

To address these questions, we analyzed data from 140 patients, who were interviewed at six-month intervals in 1992 and 1993. These data were collected as part of a study to develop alternative methods of functional status assessment (Rapkin et al., 1994). One of the approaches we developed, the Ideographic Functional Status Assessment (IFSA), started with a delineation of patients' personal goals, so that we could determine the activities and behaviors they were using to obtain their goals (Dumont, Rapkin, Smith, Correa, Palmer, & Cohen, 1999; Rapkin et al., 1994). The availability of qualitative goal assessments at two points in time, as well as several measures of health status, life events, and QOL, made it possible to analyze these data to address issues of response shifts in QOL appraisal related to personal goals. Each variable in this study may be mapped onto the response shift model presented in chapter 1.

Measures

Personal goals and response shift types. In the initial interview we used the IFSA for a 15-minute structured interview to collect data on personal goals and goal attainment activities. This analysis focuses on data from the first section of the interview, pertaining to the delineation of personal goals. The goal delineation section is divided into five major sections. Each section begins with a question about the things an individual wants to do to have the most satisfying life possible. Each section taps a different motivational orientation, phrased as follows:

1. What are the main things you want to accomplish?
2. What problems facing you do you want to solve?
3. What things do you want to prevent or avoid?
4. What things do you want to keep pretty much the same as they are now?
5. What commitments do you want to let go of?

Interviewers were trained to assist participants in phrasing their responses to these questions as a *goal statement*, which was defined as a sentence beginning with the stem "I want to . . . ", which is then completed by the respondent. After each goal statement, the interviewers probed for additional goals by asking whether there was anything else the patient wanted to accomplish, solve, and so forth.

To examine changes in personal goals over time, we modified the IFSA for the six-month follow-up. To begin this follow-up interview, we asked patients about each of the goals they had mentioned in our first interview. After providing an update on their Time 1 (T1) goals, patients were asked to identify additional, new goals that they had added since the initial interview. These new goals were elicited with the same five content probes used in the first interview (i.e., "Is there anything new you would like to accomplish?" "Any new problems you would like to solve?"). The follow-up IFSA also probed goal-attainment activity.

Goal statements were classified into eight mutually exclusive categories: global health; practical lifestyle and daily functioning; family, friends, and interpersonal relations; psychological and spiritual well-being; personal attainment and self-expression; utilizing systems and coping with society at large; altruism and societal contributions; and death and dying. Goals were sorted into these categories by a panel of raters who independently categorized each goal statement and then collaborated in resolving disagreements in classification. Eight binary variables were used to indicate whether or not patients added at least one new goal in each of the goal content categories during the six months between assessments.

Health-related QOL. The 20-item version of the Medical Outcomes Study Short-Form General Health Survey (SF-20) was administered at both times to assess health-related QOL. The instrument has been extensively used in many populations and has been shown to have good reliability and validity (Stewart, Hayes, & Ware, 1988; Wachtel et al., 1992). The SF-20 includes six subscales: physical functioning, role functioning, social functioning, mental and emotional functioning, pain, and perceptions of overall health. Given the intercorrelations among the MOS subscales, ranging from .25 to .62, principal-components analysis was conducted to further reduce these data. This approach has the advantage of parsing QOL variance into statistically orthogonal and conceptually distinct dimensions. Thus, tests for response shift effects associated with these derived dimensions are independent.

Although conducted independently, component structure loadings were virtually identical at T1 and T2 (only T1 results are presented). To account for all six MOS subscales, three unrotated components were retained, which accounted for 78% of the total variance in the MOS scales. Because orthogonal, unrotated components were retained, variance associated with all prior components was effectively removed from each later component. Thus, the first component accounted for 52.4% of the variance in MOS scales and was interpreted as global well-being. The second component, relative mental and emotional well-being, accounted for 14.3% of the variance. A high score on this component indicates that an individual's emotional well-being is high relative to others with similar levels of global well-being. Similarly, the third component accounted for 11.3% of the variance and was interpreted as relative pain. A high score here indicates that the individual's level of pain was high relative to others with similar levels of well-being.

Health status changes and life events: Catalysts of response shift. Physical symptoms were assessed at initial and follow-up interviews using a 64-item checklist of AIDS illness- and treatment-related symptoms adapted from the Health Assessment Questionnaire (Lubeck & Fries, 1994). The list was modified to include symptoms associated with AIDS in women. Symptom change over time was characterized by deriving the number of symptoms that emerged between interviews, worsened, stayed the same, improved, and disappeared. We also used a checklist of 10 common opportunistic infections to determine the number of conditions that emerged, persisted, or improved from initial to follow-up time points.

In addition to changes related to disease progression, patients were also asked about the occurrence of 30 stressful life events during the six-month interval between interviews, with a modified version of the Holmes and Rahe (1967) Social Readjustment Rating Scale. For analytic purposes, events were tallied into nine categories: death/illness of loved one, personal illness or injury, legal and drug problems, family events and household changes, problems in intimate relationships, relationship changes, economic decline, taking on new roles and responsibilities, and taking steps to care for oneself.

Demographic factors: Antecedents to response shifts. Several demographic and background variables were included to explore patient characteristics associated with change in personal goals. These included gender, age, race/ethnicity, partner status, HIV risk factors, and site of care. We also considered baseline health status and personal goal content as potential antecedents to changes in goals.

Supportive and coping resources: Potential confounds of response shift effects. As was noted earlier, changes in personal goals could lead patients to mobilize coping resources, which could in turn serve to account for change in QOL unrelated to response shifts. Although such confounds are not represented in the Sprangers and Schwartz model, it seemed necessary to take potential coping behaviors related to goals into account. Thus, several measures of change in coping resources and behavior were included in these analyses to rule out their influence on QOL before testing response shift effects. These included (a) change in the number of formal and informal sources of support (assessed at each assessment in terms of the number of network members in each category identified as providing assistance to the patient); (b) service utilization over the past six months in the following categories: hospitalizations, home nursing care, case management, mental health services, substance abuse treatment, self-help groups, legal assistance, help with housing, religious involvements, and volunteer work; and (c) change in the number of goal attainment activities associated with goals mentioned on the IFSA (see Dumont et al., 1999) for a more in-depth discussion of findings involving these scales).

Results

Demographic characteristics. The majority of participants in this study were men (87.2%) ranging in age from 24 to 66. Just under half of the respondents were ethnic minorities, including 28.1% African American and 15.4% Latino. Educational level was mixed, with nearly 25% of the sample never having completed high school, whereas 17% were college graduates. Income was low, with 70% of respondents earning less than $200 per week. Nearly two thirds of respondents were never married, and only 8.5% were married at the time of our interview, although 40.6% reported having a current main partner. More than half of the participants lived alone.

Baseline health status. In terms of health status, everyone in our sample met AIDS-defining criteria. Patients told us that they had had AIDS for two–three years on average, although 25.9% either could not recall when AIDS was diagnosed or would not describe themselves as having AIDS. All respondents reported being HIV positive, with more than 25% being diagnosed five or more years earlier, contrasted with nearly 15% being diagnosed within the past year. In terms of how people thought they were exposed to HIV, having sex with infected men was the most prevalent reason for both men (60.6%) and women (80.0%). One third of the men and two thirds of the women also listed sharing needles as a risk factor.

Changes in health status. As might be expected in a sample with advanced AIDS, numerous changes in both symptoms and AIDS-related diagnoses occurred during the six-month interval between T1 and T2. Rather than creating gross summary scales, we used separate variables to capture aspects of health status that worsened, improved, or remained the same. Indeed, many respondents experienced a mix of both positive and negative changes in their physical health. At T1, respondents reported an average of 26 out of the list of 64 physical symptoms. At follow-up, an average of 7 symptoms persisted at the same frequency over the six-month interval, whereas 4 worsened, 5 improved, and about 10 were no longer reported as problems. In addition, patients reported nearly 7 new symptoms at T2 that were not mentioned at T1. In terms of diagnoses, respondents indicated a T1 average of nearly 3 out of 26 possible opportunistic infections and other AIDS-related illnesses. At T2, respondents continued to report about a third of these diagnoses as persistent problems, whereas two thirds were no longer mentioned. However, respondents also reported an average of slightly less than one new diagnosis at T2. Consistent with the different patterns of change in health status evident in this sample, about half (54.7%) of respondents endorsed life event items, indicating that they had experienced new health problems or had gotten sicker over the past six months.

Life events. Respondents also reported high rates of non-health-related life events, including illness or death of a family member (64.7%), relationship problems (40.3%), and financial or employment problems (35.3%). In addition, 65.5% of the patients described significant changes in their household or level of contact with family, and 35.3% made changes in relationships with partners such as cohabitation. A large proportion of the sample (82.0%) reported having taken steps to care for themselves by reducing demands and entering drug treatment or other programs. Nearly one third (31.7%) reported having assumed new roles and responsibilities.

Baseline goal content. On average, people mentioned about 8 goals, ranging from 1 to 22. At baseline, patients offered an average of 1–2 goals in response to each of the five IFSA probes, with a range of 2.4 achievement-oriented goals to .75 disengagement goals. Based on our preliminary content analysis, people's goals covered a wide range of concerns. Goals related to practical living situations and daily functioning were most common, with nearly 2 such goals mentioned on average. Concerns for health and for family and friends were also prevalent. Other issues came up more sporadically, including altruism, death and dying, and societal problems. Patients' responses across these 8 areas of concern were almost completely independent (correlations ranged from $r = -.15$ to $r = .19$, with only 3 areas significant). In other words, individuals who were likely to mention goals in one category were no more or less likely to mention goals in other content categories. This variety in content and patterning of personal goals speaks to the many frames of reference that people use to appraise their QOL.

Changes in goal content. On average, patients mentioned 1.4 additional goals that were not of concern at T1. There were marked individual differences in the number of goals added: 22.0% of respondents stated that they had not added any new goals since T1, whereas 39.7% mentioned 1 new goal, 26.2% mentioned 2 new goals, and 12.0% mentioned 3–6 new goals. New goals were distributed across different areas of concern. Table 4.1 summarizes the proportion of patients who mentioned goals in each goal content category at T1, as well as the proportion who added goals by category at T2. New goals tended to involve daily demands, personal growth, and interpersonal relationships. General health goals were some-

Table 4.1. Changes in Goals on the Ideographic Functional Status Assessment Among 140 AIDS Patients

IFSA Goal Content Category	% naming at least one goal at Time 1	% adding at least one goal at Time 2
Global health	90.0	20.6
Daily demands	87.9	20.6
Interpersonal	72.9	24.8
Emotional well-being	58.6	12.8
Personal growth	47.1	25.5
Altruism	31.4	2.8
Systems barriers	28.6	6.4
Death and dying	18.6	4.3

Note. IFSA = Ideographic Functional Status Assessment.

what less prevalent, as were goals related to emotional well-being. Relatively few participants added goals related to system barriers, altruism, or death and dying. Although it does not appear that patients completely revised their personal goals between T1 and T2, many did take on new goals in one or several life domains. This information made it possible to determine whether and how response shifts in QOL were associated with these relatively subtle changes in priorities and concerns.

Antecedents of changes in goals. Hierarchical logistic regression analyses were conducted to explore characteristics associated with the addition of new goals in each category. Variables entered included demographic characteristics; T1 measures of health status, QOL, and personal goals; and changes in health status and life events. There were relatively few relationships between demographic factors and changes in goals (see Table 4.2). Most notably, women were more likely to add interpersonal and emotional well-being goals. Ethnic minorities were more likely to emphasize interpersonal goals and less likely to mention daily demands. Patients with better initial QOL tended to pursue new health-related or daily-demand goals. Patients in poorer health but with relatively high mental functioning focused on personal growth. Alternatively, more goals related to preparation for death and dying were reported by patients who were sicker at T1, who had experienced financial or employment-related problems, and who did not have to deal with the illness of a loved one.

Detection of response shifts in QOL associated with changes in personal goals. As has been discussed, hierarchical regression analysis may be used to determine whether residual variance in QOL change scores (after controlling for health status changes and other life events) can be explained by interaction effects associated with personal goals. These interactions indicate that health status changes or other events (i.e., catalysts in the Sprangers and Schwartz model) have a different impact on the QOL of

Table 4.2. Antecedents of Goal Changes on the Ideographic Functional Status Assessment Among 140 AIDS Patients

IFSA Goal Content Category	OR
Global health	
High initial mental functioning	1.87**
Few interpersonal goals	0.67*
Daily demands	
Who are not ethnic minority	0.38*
High initial global functioning	1.49*
More initial personal-growth goals	1.56*
More persistent symptoms	1.05*
Making changes to reduce load	1.57*
Interpersonal	
Female	3.35*
Ethnic minority	3.92**
Personal growth	
High initial opportunistic infections	1.23*
High initial mental functioning	1.52
High initial relative pain	1.77**
Few illness-related events	0.60*
Emotional well-being	
Being female	3.22
Altruistic	
Persistent opportunistic infections	3.60**
Increased responsibilities	5.20**
Systems barriers	
High initial personal growth goals	1.86*
Taking on new roles	2.26*
Death and dying	
High initial opportunistic infections	1.45*
Low initial global functioning	0.33*
High initial interpersonal goals	1.83*
Not experiencing illness or death of loved one	0.14
Loss of economic security	4.94*

Note. IFSA = Ideographic Functional Status Assessment, $^{*}p < .05$. $^{**}p < .01$.

people who added particular types of goals compared to those who did not change their goals in that way.

The potential number of interaction terms that are involved in examining how various changes in goals moderate the impact of different catalysts is quite large. Several steps were taken to limit the number of interactions tested and to avoid capitalizing on chance. First, additional goals in low prevalence categories (altruism, system barriers, death and dying) were not considered in response shift analyses. Second, separate initial regression analyses were conducted to test all interaction effects associated with each of the five remaining categories of goal changes for each of the three QOL variables. Third, only interaction effects significant at $p < .05$ in initial analysis were retained for subsequent analysis. Fourth, after significant interaction terms associated with each type of goal change were identified, they were entered together in a final summary analysis for each QOL component. This made it possible to account for potential multicolinearity in the moderator effects (for example, if a shift toward either daily-demand goals or health goals produced similar, correlated response shifts in attenuating the impact of declining health on global well-being). Fifth, possible confounds associated with the mobilization of support and coping resources were entered into the regression prior to response shift moderators. Sixth, by using orthogonal component scores, analyses associated with each of the different QOL outcomes are nonredundant. Results of the three summary regression models are presented in Table 4.3.

Change in global well-being. After controlling for 16% of the variance in change that was due to initial functioning, an additional 31% of the variance could be explained by changes in health status. Non-health-related life events were not associated with this component, indicating that the largest component of QOL variance in this sample is specifically related to changes in health status. Pursuit of new personal-growth goals had a small but significant positive impact on global well-being in this sample (1% of variance), as did the related coping resources associated with religious and volunteer involvements (4% of variance). Together, these influences accounted for 51% of the variance of change in global well-being.

After all other effects were controlled, goal-by-catalyst interactions accounted for 8% of the variance of change in global well-being. Three distinct response shift effects were evident. Patients who had increased health concerns experienced more pronounced negative reactions to illness or injuries over the past six months. In contrast, these patients seemed to be less affected by disruptions in family and household routine. In addition, persistent symptoms had a more negative impact on appraisals of global functioning among patients who were attempting to pursue new personal-growth goals.

Emotional well-being and mental functioning. Emotional well-being at T1 accounted for 27% of the variance in change in emotional well-being. Worsening symptoms were associated with declines in emotional well-being. This effect became slightly more pronounced when we controlled for the correlation between symptoms and the emergence of new opportunistic infections (a suppression effect), such that health status changes accounted for 7% of change in emotional well-being. Non-health-related life events, specifically legal and substance-use related problems, accounted for another 6% of the variance. Use of legal services offset this decrease somewhat, accounting for another 2% increment in R^2. Together, initial status, health changes, life events, and coping resources accounted for 40% of the variance of change in emotional well-being.

At the final step of the regression model, goal-by-catalyst interaction effects accounted for an additional 6% of the variance associated with change in relative emotional well-being and mental functioning. These findings suggest that patients who adopted new personal-growth goals benefited more from reductions in symptoms, whereas those who concentrated on new daily demands benefited less. Again, these interaction effects were strengthened when we took into account a suppression effect involving improvement in opportunistic infections, indicating that it was specifically symptom relief, not change in diagnoses, that fostered improved emotional well-being among patients pursuing new personal-growth goals.

Relative pain. After controlling for 46% of the variance related to initial pain, increase in relative pain was uncorrelated with changes in health status and non-health-related life events. This lack of relationship suggests that principal-components analysis succeeded in isolating distinct components of QOL. However, this negative finding raised the question as to whether this component was picking up meaningful variation in QOL or merely random error. In fact, change in relative pain was significantly associated with several indicators of goal change and coping, including pursuing new personal-growth goals (2% of the variance), increases in religious participation (1%), and goal attainment activities (3%). Interestingly, increases in these goals and coping efforts were associated with greater pain, suggesting that pain was more disruptive for these patients. All told, these effects accounted for 52% of the variance.

As with emotional well-being, two types of goal-by-catalyst interactions were significantly associated with pain, related to daily-demands goals and personal-growth goals. These accounted for 7% of the variance of change in relative pain and suggested several kinds of response shifts. Similar to the emotional well-being component, people who took on new personal-growth goals reported reduced pain in the face of persistent illness. Consistent with the interpretation of the main effects, pain was more pronounced among patients who took on new role responsibilities apparently linked to new personal-growth goals. Similarly, ratings of pain were more pronounced among patients who were pursuing new daily-demand goals in the context of changes in family roles and household routines. Alternatively, pain ratings decreased for people who were able to take more care of themselves and lighten their load while pursuing new daily-demand goals.

Relative magnitude of response shift effects. It is worth noting that goal-by-catalyst interaction effects accounted for approximately the same proportion of variance on each of the three, independent components of change in QOL (between 6% and 8%). Although this may be coincidental, it does suggest that health-related, emotional, and "disruptive pain" dimensions of QOL are equally subject to response shift effects. From another perspective, the relative importance of response shift effects increased across the three analyses. For successive components, the ratios of variance that were due to response shifts to total variance explained by effects other than initial status were .08/.43, .06/.19, and .07/.13—or 18.6%, 31.6%, and 53.8%, respectively. After controlling for major effects associated with gross changes in health status, QOL response shifts apparently become even more pronounced. Sources of variance in QOL

Table 4.3. Regressions Predicting Change in the Quality-of-Life Components

Effects in the model	Global well-being			Relative emotional			Relative pain		
	r	∃z	R^2	r	∃z	R^2	r	∃z	R^2
Baseline-level health status	−0.40***	−0.47***	0.16***	−0.52***	−0.54***	0.27***	−0.68***	−0.65***	0.46***
			0.31***			0.07**			0.00
Symptoms									
Abated	0.41***	0.11$^+$		0.00			−0.02		
Improved	0.10			0.01			−0.01		
Persisted	−0.19*			−0.10			0.08		
Worsened	−0.28**	−0.19**		−0.20*	−0.27***		0.05		
Emerged	−0.34***			0.02			0.06		
Infections									
Abated	0.27**			−0.07			−0.05		
Persisted	−0.04	−0.24***		0.08	0.13$^+$		−0.02		
Emerged	−0.30***			0.05			−0.02		
Illness or Injury	−0.34***	−0.21**		−0.08			0.17$^+$		
Life events			0.00			0.06***			0.00
Death or illness of loved one	−0.01			−0.05			−0.05		
Legal and drug problems	−0.10			−0.20*	−0.27***		0.06		
Relationship problems	−0.11			0.07			0.10		
Money problems	0.04			−0.01			0.11		
Relationship changes	−0.01			−0.02			0.01		
Family changes	0.06			0.00			0.15$^+$		
New roles	0.09			−0.11			−0.01		
Lightening load, off drugs	−0.16$^+$			−0.11			0.00		
Change in personal goals			0.01$^+$			0.00			0.02*
General health	0.15$^+$			−0.08			0.17*		
Interpersonal	−0.07			0.01			0.15$^+$		

Emotional	0.02			−0.05			0.03		
Personal growth	0.20*	0.29**		0.03			−0.10	0.07	
Daily demands	−0.14			−0.09			−0.06		
Coping resources			0.04**			0.02^{+}			0.01^{+}
Self-help	−0.03			0.09			−0.13		
Legal services	−0.06			0.01			0.09		
Housing assistance	0.02			0.16^{+}			−0.05		
Religious organizations	0.18*	0.17**		0.10			0.09	0.10^{+}	
Volunteer work	0.11	0.10^{+}		−0.08			−0.03		
Goal attainment activities response shift effects	0.13		0.00	−0.02		0.00	0.19*	0.18**	0.03**
			0.08***			0.06**			0.07***
Health goals									
With family changes	0.24**	0.31***		−0.09			0.27***		
With illness or injury	−0.02	−0.18*		−0.06			0.19*		
Personal-growth goals									
With persistent symptoms	0.02	−0.21*		−0.08			−0.02		
With abated symptoms	0.29***			0.12	0.25**		−0.07		
With abated infections	0.19*			−0.08	−0.20*		−0.06		
With persistent infections	0.09			0.04			−0.11	−0.14*	
With new roles	−0.05			−0.11			0.07	0.16*	
Daily demand goals									
With abated symptoms	0.08			-0.14^{+}	-0.14^{+}		−0.07		
With lightening load, off drugs	−0.09			−0.06			−0.13	−0.25***	
With family changes	−0.11			−0.03			0.15^{+}	0.24**	
Total R^2			0.59***			0.46***			0.59***

Note. $^{+}p < 0.10$. $^{*}p < 0.05$. $^{**}p < 0.01$. $^{***}p < 0.001$.

change that are more strongly associated with response shift effects can be isolated to some extent, using principal-components analysis.

Discussion

Response shift effects in all aspects of QOL emerged, above and beyond adjustments for initial QOL, direct effects of stressors, evidence of coping (changes in goals themselves and the number of goal attainment strategies), and indicators of active coping (changes in informal and formal support, extent of use of services over the past six months in eight categories). Admittedly, these effects emerged as the result of a series of exploratory regressions. There is the possibility that our findings capitalized on sample-specific relationships. However, confidence in these results is increased by the following observations:

1. Interpretable goal-by-catalyst interaction effects emerged in analyses with three distinct and orthogonal QOL scales.
2. Although stepwise criteria were used to enter response shift variables, they were also used to enter direct effects of coping indicators. Response shift effects typically equaled or exceeded the variance explained by other predictors.
3. All other predictors were entered at the $p < .10$ level, whereas response shift interactions were allowed to enter only at the $p < .05$ level. Note that these effects emerged despite the inherent statistical problems in detecting multiplicative interactions using regression analysis (McClelland, 1993).
4. Response shifts related to different types of goals tended to add to variance explained rather than overlap.

Furthermore, it is noteworthy that these results emerged in a fairly homogeneous sample of adults living with AIDS for an average of three years. All were already linked to networks of care, receiving multiple services and being treated for one or more opportunistic infections. If anything, it should be more difficult to detect important changes in goals and related response shifts among people who have had many years to accommodate to an illness. Even so, changes in physical health status and stressful life events still demonstrated both direct effects on QOL and effects moderated by response shifts. Indeed, even reactions to prolonged problems related to chronic illness (i.e., persistent symptoms) were subject to response shifts.

Most important, response shift effects were interpretable, and they could be readily understood in terms of the phenomenology of a person living with AIDS. For example, patients who placed increased emphasis on a general desire to get better seemed to be less affected by non-health-related events but were more strongly affected by disease progression. Although pursuing personal-growth goals seemed to help patients cope with ongoing problems, pursuing these goals also led patients to report greater disruption or distress associated with pain. Patients who placed more emphasis on meeting day-to-day demands reported relatively greater improvement in QOL when they could reduce responsibilities and obligations and care for themselves, and greater decrement in QOL when new roles led to increased responsibilities. Patients who shifted their focus toward meeting daily demands were also less likely to enjoy the benefits of reduced symptoms.

In summary, these findings suggest four kinds of response shifts related to changes in personal goals and concerns. Specifically, patients tended to

1. have more positive reactions to events that made obtaining goals more likely
2. have more negative reactions to events that directly interfered with obtaining goals
3. have attenuated reactions to positive and negative events that were less directly relevant to goal attainment
4. have different reactions to emergent versus entrenched health problems, depending on the implications of health problems for goal attainment.

These findings point to several important directions for further research. The first is to develop a more detailed description of change in personal goals. In this analysis, changes in goals were treated as distinct and separable events. In fact, it may be more accurate to describe shifts in goal content in terms of patterns of change in goals. For example, the implications of a shift toward global health concerns may depend on whether the individual is moving away from interpersonal concerns or personal-growth concerns. Of course, individuals may increase their concerns in several domains at once. It would be interesting to determine whether simultaneous increases in both the personal-growth and interpersonal domains prove to have complementary benefits or are mutually antagonistic, in terms of the appraisal of long-standing problems and new crises. It may also be important to determine the magnitude of a response shift. In our analysis, goal shifts were measured with binary indicators (were one or more goals added in a given area?). A small number of individuals added multiple goals in one or more areas. It is unclear whether the same response shift effects would simply be more pronounced in these individuals or whether other effects might emerge. All of these issues could be explored with the methodology introduced in this study, although a much larger sample size would be required.

More in-depth goal content assessment would shed light on additional aspects of response shift. In this analysis, personal goals were coded only in terms of broad content areas. Content analysis could describe other aspects of personal goals, including motivational orientation (achievement, maintenance, disengagement), level of aspiration (high demand versus low demand on self or resources), specificity of objectives, time frame involved in goal attainment, and disease relevance. These dimensions may not be independent. For example, daily-demand goals may be more specific and involve problem solving, whereas interpersonal goals may be more open-ended and focused on maintaining relationships. This suggests the need to describe attributes of personal goals in terms of underlying content dimensions.

There are also several limitations inherent in the ideographic assessment methodology used in this research. Although ideographic methods allow individuals to identify their most salient goals, there is no guarantee that this method is sufficiently thorough in probing all aspects of motivation. It is also difficult to ensure that individuals consider similar levels in a goal hierarchy using ideographic methods. For instance, one person may say that he wants to "see his family more," whereas another may say that she wants to "see her parents this weekend." It is not clear whether or how such differences in goal content matter in understanding response shifts. Nomothetic assessment of goal content through the use of an inventory might help offset this problem, because individuals are prompted to consider a wide range of alternative goals, yielding scores on key goal attribute dimensions (Rapkin & Fischer, 1992). Ideally, ideographic and nomothetic techniques might be administered together to provide a more complete assessment.

An inherent problem in understanding changes in goals and their impact on self-reports of QOL involves the distinction between coping and response shifts. It is probably the case that emotion-focused coping utilizes changes in goals to reduce the impact of threats and losses. Response shifts are inextricably involved with this aspect of coping, and it makes the most sense to understand all changes in goals as having the potential to attenuate threats. Of course, goal change is also involved in problem-focused coping, leading the individual to pursue or maintain supports and resources or to try new avenues for satisfaction. In our analysis, we controlled for the number of goal attainment strategies and for other evidence of attempts at problem-focused coping, including mobilization of services and supports. Unfortunately, relying on these statistical controls may be too conservative, potentially obscuring response shift effects. For example, the appraisal that new support is available may in part depend on goal-based response shifts concerning what constitutes relevant support.

The study described in this chapter demonstrates that people's goals and concerns continue to change during the course of serious illness, perhaps to the end of life. These changes in priorities and perspectives influence the ways in which individuals react to illness and other stressors, as is evidenced by differences in responses to questions about their QOL. Deeper understanding of changes in personal goals and their relationship to response shifts in QOL will require further theoretical formulation of the underlying mechanisms. However, to achieve a truly humanistic and patient-centered approach to research and practice, it is essential to pay close attention to the goals that matter most to each individual throughout illness and treatment.

References

Andrews, F. M., & Withey, S. B. (1976). *Social indicators of well-being: Americans' perceptions of life quality*. New York: Plenum Press.

Bühler, C., Brind, A., & Horner, A. (1968). Old age as a phase of human life. *Human Development, 11*, 53–63.

Calman, K. C. (1984). The quality of life in cancer patients—an hypothesis. *Journal of Medical Ethics, 10*, 124–127.

Campbell, A., Converse, P. E., & Rodgers W. L. (1976). *The quality of American life*. New York: Russell Sage Foundation.

Cantril, H. (1965). *The pattern of human concerns*. New Brunswick, NJ: Rutgers University Press.

Cella, D. F., & Tulsky, D. S. (1990). Measuring quality of life today: Methodological aspects. *Oncology, 4*(5), 29–39.

De Haes, J. C. J. M., & van Knippenberg, F. C. E. (1987). Quality of life of cancer patients: Review of the literature. In N. K. Aaronson & J. H. Beckmann (Eds.), *The quality of life of cancer patients* (pp. 167–182). New York: Raven Press.

Diener, E. (1984). Subjective well-being. *Psychological Bulletin, 95*, 542–575.

Dumont K. A., Rapkin, B. D., Smith, M. Y., Correa, A., Palmer, S., & Cohen, S. (1999). The relationship between health and human services and the personal goal-directed activities of persons living with AIDS. *American Journal of Community Psychology, 27*(7), 55–73.

Emmons, R. (1986). Personal strivings: An approach to personality and subjective well-being. *Journal of Personality and Social Psychology, 51*, 1058–1068.

George, L. K., & Bearon, L. B. (1980). *Quality of life in older persons: Meaning and measurement*. New York: Human Sciences Press.

Holmes, T. H., & Rahe, R. H. (1967). The social readjustment scale. *Journal of Psychosomatic Research, 11*, 213–218.

Klinger, E., Barta, S. G., & Maxleiner, M. E. (1980). Motivational correlates of thought content frequency and commitment. *Journal of Personality and Social Psychology, 39*, 1222–1237.

Lubeck D. P., & Fries, J. F. (1994). Changes in health status after one year for persons at-risk for and with HIV infection. *Psychology and Health, 9*, 79–92.

McClelland, G. H. (1993). Statistical difficulties of detecting interactions and moderator effects. *Psychological Bulletin, 114*, 376–390.

Morris, J. N., & Sherwood, S. (1987). Quality of life of cancer patients at different stages in the disease trajectory. *Journal of Chronic Diseases, 40*, 545–553.

Palys, T. S., & Little, B. R. (1983). Perceived life satisfaction and the organization of personal project systems. *Journal of Personality and Social Psychology, 44*, 1221–1230.

Rapkin, B. D., & Fischer, K. (1992). Personal goals of older adults: Issues in assessment and prediction. *Psychology and Aging, 7*(1), 127–137.

Rapkin, B. D., Smith, M. Y., Dumont, K., Correa, A., Palmer, S., & Cohen, S. (1994). Development of the ideographic functional status assessment: A measure of the personal goals and goal attainment of people with AIDS. *Psychology and Health, 9*, 111–129.

Sartorius, N. (1987) Cross-cultural comparisons of data about quality of life: A sample of issues. In N. K. Aaronson & J. H. Beckmann (Eds.), *The quality of life of cancer patients* (pp. 19–24). New York: Raven Press.

Schipper, H., Clinch, J., McMurray, A., & Levitt, M. (1984). Measuring quality of life of cancer patients. The Functional Living Index-Cancer: Development and validation. *Journal of Clinical Oncology, 2*, 472–483.

Stewart, A. L., Hays, R. D., & Ware, J. E. (1988). The MOS Short-form General Health Survey: Reliability and validity in a patient population. *Medical Care, 26*(7), 724–732.

Wachtel, T., Piette, J., Mor, V., Stein, M., Fleishman, J., & Carpenter, C. (1992). Quality of life in persons with human immunodeficiency virus infection: Measurement by the Medical Outcomes Study instrument. *Annals of Internal Medicine, 116*(2), 129–137.

5

Discussion: Theoretical Reflections

Carolyn E. Schwartz
and Mirjam A. G. Sprangers

Response shift highlights three distinct aspects of change—in internal standards, values, and conceptualization—that are currently below the surface of measurement. By making response shift explicit, it is expected that our understanding of how humans experience change will be advanced. The maturation of any new construct depends on a strong theoretical foundation that links the new construct to existing concepts, guides hypothesis generation, and directs the creation of new measures. The chapters in this part of the book, "Theoretical Reflections," have addressed the theoretical foundation of response shift. In this discussion chapter, we summarize the advances represented by the foregoing chapters and highlight the intricacies that have yet to be clarified.

In chapter 1, we propose a theoretical model to explain the presence or absence of response shift as a result of a catalyst and the interaction of antecedents and mechanisms. Whereas *antecedents* refer to stable characteristics of the individual, *mechanisms* entail behavioral, cognitive, and affective processes to adjust to the catalytic health state change. The interaction of antecedents and mechanisms leads to response shifts, which are postulated to affect perceived quality of life (QOL). The other chapters in this part address and expand the theoretical framework for response shift phenomena in various populations and regarding different antecedents and mechanisms. Richards and Folkman (chapter 2) address response shifts among bereaved caregivers from a coping perspective. In chapter 3, Lepore and Eton compare the fit of suppressor and buffering models by using data that operationalize recalibration and reprioritization response shifts in prostate cancer patients. Rapkin (chapter 4) focuses on how goal setting and changes in goals over the course of disease elicit reprioritization response shift and how this inclusion of response shift explains more variance in perceived QOL. Thus each chapter confronts some of the conceptual intricacies of the model.

This work was supported in part by the Agency for Health Care Policy and Research, Grant 1 RO1 HSO-8582-03 to Carolyn E. Schwartz.

We thank Ivan Barofsky and Bruce Rapkin for helpful discussions.

Conceptualization Issues

In the time since the theoretical model was first conceptualized, a number of questions have emerged that merit some discussion. The first set of questions concern the conceptualization of response shift, in particular the interdependence of its components. It is debatable the extent to which changes in internal standards, values, and conceptualization should be expected to shift equivalently and in parallel. For example, if changes in internal standards of fatigue suggest the use of a lower anchoring point, would that imply that the same anchor refers to a different experience of fatigue—that is, a reconceptualization of fatigue? Would it imply changes in the importance of being tired relative to other related QOL domains, such as pain, social functioning, or mood? Future research should elucidate the underlying conceptual links between the aspects of response shift.

In addition to conceptual issues raised in this part of the book regarding the adaptiveness and consciousness of response shift, another issue that merits attention is whether response shift is an active or passive process. For example, patients might *engage in* response shift or merely may *undergo* response shift, the latter implying that it happens without choice or forethought. It may be that it is characterized by both active and passive processes depending on the context. Accordingly, the conditions that differentiate the type of process need to be elucidated. This question has particular implications for interventions that might teach response shift, because teaching what is normally a passive process may require different approaches than may teaching what is normally an active process. It also has consequences for assessment strategies, because more active processes might be more amenable to direct, self-report measurement, whereas passive processes may require inferential assessment strategies or statistical modeling.

Issues About the Model Itself

Another set of questions concerns the interconnectedness between components of the model. If one is unclear how mechanisms or outcomes are distinct from response shift, then the benefit of the construct becomes refutable. This problem becomes apparent in several contexts. First, there is a logical circularity introduced if the operationalization of a mechanism is synonymous with the operationalization of response shift. For example, goal reordering is posited as a mechanism that would lead to reprioritization and perhaps reconceptualization. If one measures reported goals and their changing importance status, then is one measuring the mechanism or the response shift? Rapkin resolves this issue by distinguishing the measurement of goals (i.e., the mechanism) from the statistical operationalization of response shift (i.e., interaction effects of changes in goals with the impact of disease progression, life events, or treatments on QOL). This distinction in the operationalization of mechanism and response shift facilitates the continued development of response shift theory and measurement.

A second circularity becomes apparent when the process of response shift becomes synonymous with the outcome of response shift. This problem is similar to one faced by researchers of coping in cases where the process of coping became synonymous with the outcome of coping. For example, effective copers might use more problem-solving strategies in controllable situations, which may result in the resolution of the problem. Likewise, lowering one's internal standards, an aspect of response shift, might be seen as a reframing coping strategy or as the outcome of that process. Accordingly, at the level of measurement we can see an overlap between response shift and the QOL outcome. For example, if QOL is assessed solely with a questionnaire that is being used simultaneously to assess changes in internal standards, then these two components may not be distinguishable (e.g., the thentest procedure). This possible overlap reflects a conceptual dilemma that needs to be clarified.

A third context in which this circularity may be problematic is inherent in the early phase of new construct development. One must tease apart the validity of a measure (i.e., Do two measures of the same aspect of response shift identify similar shifts in direction, magnitude, domain?) from the validity of the construct (i.e., Are the three components of response shift empirically linked?). This challenge may be resolved iteratively as one implements studies that include several approaches to measuring a response shift component. Once concurrent validity is established for measures of the three components of response shift, then one can empirically test the validity of the construct using structural equation modeling on larger (e.g., N = 200) study samples followed over time.

Definitional Issues

There are two components of the model that require consideration and development: the catalysts and mechanisms of response shift. According to the Sprangers and Schwartz model, changes in one's own health state act as catalytic events of response shifts. Whereas Rapkin examines response shifts in goals as a function of health state change, Lepore and Eton test response shift hypotheses by comparing patients with stable or deteriorating health states to patients whose health state has improved. In chapter 9, Sprangers et al. compare patients who improve with those who deteriorate and drop stable patients from the analysis. These variations in grouping patients may yield findings that are not comparable to each other. Future researchers might consider collecting data in which response shift is measured explicitly and examining whether and how the phenomena differ among patients whose health state has deteriorated, remained stable, or improved.

A second consideration in the definition of catalyst is that it is conceivable that changes in a loved one's health state or even the mere passage of time may induce changes in internal standards, values, or conceptualization. Richards and Folkman illustrate how changes in a loved one's health and his subsequent death catalyzed response shifts via meaning-based coping processes. These processes were invoked when previous beliefs, expectations, and goals were no longer tenable. That the mere passage of time may invoke response shift may render it difficult to predict under what circumstances response shift will take place. It would thus be useful to attempt to define other parameters of life or time that are relevant and likely to differentiate people who are expected to undergo response shift. This line of investigation might be facilitated, for example, by qualitative methods that query cognitive processing. Envisioning the passage of time as a catalyst has repercussions on study design and data analysis. For example, longitudinal studies with standardized data collection intervals may obscure the presence of response shift effects. Accordingly, one might investigate alternative research designs whereby the data collection intervals are individually tailored to capture the active period of response shifting. The recent availability of statistical techniques that do not require identical intervals or similar follow-up across participants may be particularly useful in this regard. These types of methods will prove increasingly useful as the questions integral to response shift development become more identified.

Another component of the model that will require consideration and development is mechanisms. One notable conceptual challenge concerns the difficulty of creating appropriate scores to operationalize a given mechanism. For example, one can measure spiritual practice habits over several points in time. The question that arises is how to combine these data points to reflect the mechanism of spiritual practice. Should one simply examine relationships among model components at each singular point in time? Or should one use lagged models, where early reports of spiritual practice habits are used to predict later scores of response shift and outcome? Alternatively, one might consider other frameworks that model change in either the level or rate of spiritual practice over time. On a conceptual level, the approaches modeling change in level or rate are more consistent with the underlying dynamics postulated by response shift theory. As response shift data are collected in larger samples of patients, the differential advantages of these and other approaches to operationalizing mechanisms can be investigated.

Conclusion

In this discussion we have addressed some of the intricacies inherent in the development of the response shift construct. These conceptual issues include the potential circularity of this early stage in construct development, the problem of confounding model components and operationalization of response shifts, the implications of grouping people with regard to the likelihood of engaging in response shifts for the purpose of hypothesis testing, and the issue of identifying relevant catalysts. Although these issues represent important caveats that must be considered as investigators proceed in the empirical study of the construct, they also provide exciting and promising directions for future research. The next part of the book builds on the theoretical foundation provided in this first part. The contributors examine potential assessment tools for measuring response shift, possible sources of artifact that might be confused with response shift, and empirical work in which response shifts were measured using individualized methods or design approaches.

Part II

Methodological Pathways

6

Methodological Approaches for Assessing Response Shift in Longitudinal Health-Related Quality-of-Life Research

Carolyn E. Schwartz and Mirjam A. G. Sprangers

Introduction

Research on social factors and health relies heavily on the measurement of perceived quality of life (QOL). It is founded, however, on assumptions about the stability of intra-individual standards which may not be valid. As people can vary, so can their values. This variability may reflect informative shifts in an individual's internal standards, in values and priorities, or in the conceptualization of perceived QOL, in addition to changes in actual health state. This 'response shift' phenomenon is of fundamental importance to social and medical science.

As an illustration, the results of a psychosocial randomized trial (Schwartz, 1999) will be described, the objective of which was to compare the effectiveness of a coping skills group intervention as compared to a

We would like to acknowledge the invaluable contribution of the following social and medical scientists who participated in the Response Shift Workshop which was held in Boston, December 1996, and funded by Agency for Health Care Policy and Research (1 RO1 HSO8582-01A1) to CES and by a matched contribution from Frontier Science. These participants included: Achilles Armenakis, PhD; Katy Benjamin, SM, MSW; Lawren Daltroy, DPH; Susan Folkman, PhD; Rick Gibbons, PhD; Maureen Wilson Genderson, MA; Hanneke de Haes, PhD; Hang Lee, PhD; Geraldine Padilla, PhD; Allen Parducci, PhD; Bruce Rapkin, PhD; Patricia Rieker, PhD; Rabbi Meir Sendor, PhD; and Ira Wilson, MD, MSc. We are also indebted to David Mohr, PhD, Peter Vitaliano, PhD, Paul Osterveld, PhD, and Angela de Boer, PhD, for stimulating discussions about response shift; to Michael Babyak, PhD, for helpful discussions regarding growth curve analysis applications to response shift; to Hang Lee, PhD, for helpful discussions regarding algebraic formulations based on triangulated data sources; to Leslie Lenert, MD, and Peep Stalmeier, PhD, for helpful discussions about Prospect Theory; and to David Waldman, PhD, Steven Locke, MD, and Jon Treadwell, PhD, for helpful discussions about hysteresis. We would also like to thank Elisa Laitin and Amy Carey for assistance with manuscript preparation, and Achilles Armenakis, PhD, for helpful comments on an earlier draft of this manuscript.

peer telephone support intervention for people with multiple sclerosis. These results motivated a quest for methods which measure response shift. The group intervention consisted of a comprehensive package which included cognitive, behavioral and supportive techniques aimed at helping patients to accommodate to their progressive disease trajectory. The peer telephone support intervention involved less intensive contact, no in-person meetings and was non-directive. Given the chronic and non-fatal nature of this auto-immune disease, patients had a prognosis for a normal lifespan with periods of relapses and progressive disability (Lechtenberg, 1988).

Two-year follow-up data suggested that despite significant deterioration in neuropsychological performance, neurological disability and self-efficacy function, participants in the group intervention reported reduced psychosocial role limitations, decreased use of negative coping strategies and enhanced well-being. In contrast, peer support recipients did not report significant changes in psychosocial role performance, coping, or well-being. Thus, although both groups exhibited significant deterioration in clinical measures of function, the well-known disparity between patient-reported and clinical measures of function was largest in the coping skills group.

The apparent separation of physical functioning and psychological well-being may represent 'response shift phenomenon.' Our working definition of response shift refers to a change in the meaning of one's self-evaluation of a target construct as a result of: (a) a change in the respondent's internal standards of measurement (i.e. scale recalibration); (b) a change in the respondent's values (i.e. the importance of component domains constituting the target construct) or (c) a redefinition of the target construct (i.e. reconceptualization). Indeed, qualitative interviews with participants revealed that they felt that meeting people in the group who were worse or better off than they were led them to change their internal standards of how badly off they themselves were. Additionally, they felt that the group intervention helped them to reconsider the goals that were important and feasible to them (i.e. changes in values), and to learn that it was possible to have a reasonable QOL even with a worse condition (i.e. reconceptualization of QOL). This example illustrates how a psychosocial intervention might *teach* response shift.

The concept of response shift has its foundation in research on educational training interventions (Howard et al., 1979a, 1979b, 1979c, 1981) and organizational change (Golembiewski et al., 1976). Whereas Howard and colleagues defined response shift in terms of changes in internal standards of measurement, Golembiewski et al. introduced the component of changes in conceptualization and internal standards. Investigators from the discipline of management sciences described a typology of change which distinguished alpha, beta and gamma shifts, referring to objective changes, change in internal standards and reconceptualizations, respectively (Armenakis, 1988). The working definition adds changes in values as another component that is relevant to a change in the meaning of one's self-evaluation. While changes in values were inherent in the Golembiewski description of reconceptualization, the working definition adopted in this paper includes this as a separate third component that is relevant to the change in the meaning of one's self-evaluation. Making it a distinct third aspect will thus highlight its importance and emphasizes the need to measure it carefully (Sprangers & Schwartz, 1999). Finally, this working definition avoids the use of the terms 'beta' and 'gamma' shift since these terms do not reveal their content. It would be preferable to use the more transparent terms of change in internal standards, change in value and reconceptualization.

Response shift is important to consider in treatment evaluations, especially insofar as it may serve to attenuate or to exaggerate estimates of treatment effects as patients adapt to treatment toxicities or disease progression over time. Methods which assess response shift will not only be necessary to reveal unbiased treatment effects, but will also be useful for examining the impact of illness over time. The purpose of the present work is to discuss existing methods or those which can be developed to address the different components of response shift. As will be noted below, these approaches operationalize more than one aspect of response shift, a measurement challenge which may reflect an inherent inter-connection between internal standards, values and conceptualization. This interconnection will be discussed in greater depth after the methods have been presented. Our goal is to encourage and facilitate research on this construct.

Methods

Several of the methods which will be described are protocols we are suggesting for adapting existing tools so that they can assess one or more of the three aspects of response shift. Others are new methods developed by the authors and for which empirical substantiation is currently underway. Finally, we also describe approaches which would influence the design of new studies or the analysis of existing data sets. Including outcome tools, design approaches and statistical methods in the assessment battery will stimulate response shift research in cross-sectional or longitudinal research as well as secondary analyses of existing data.

These methods will be evaluated according to four criteria, including: (1) feasibility (i.e. understandability, time, and costs), (2) reliability (i.e. test–retest or internal consistency reliability), (3) validity (i.e. criterion, discriminant, content, or construct validity) and (4) whether empirical evidence is available in QOL research or other areas of research (Table 6.1). Future directions for developing each of the methods or approaches will also be outlined. As a caveat, it should be noted that this discussion may be unbalanced to the extent that some of the methods or adaptations of existing methods have little or no empirical data to support or refute their use. Consequently, it will be easier to criticize existing methods with data than new or adapted methods without.

Table 6.1. Methods for Assessing Response Shift

Method	Aspect(s) of response shift measured	Feasibility	Reliability established?	Validity established?	Empirical data available?
Individualized methods					
Repertory Grid Technique	change in values reconceptualization	baseline data must be provided at posttest; structured interviews required for all examples, therefore time-consuming; multimedia software might be useful	would be similar to reliability of original method for all examples; can be improved by sampling multiple domains as well as overall QOL	NA	NA
Cantril's Ladder	change in internal standards reconceptualization			NA	NA
SEIQoL	change in values reconceptualization			NA	NA
Preference-based methods					
Extended Q-TWiST	change in values	analytic method which is potentially time-consuming as it requires collecting data on preferences, QOL, and social cost	NR	NR	yes

Preference Mapping	change in values	potentially time-consuming and requires complex statistical methods; may be facilitated with multi-media software	NA	NA	NA
Successive comparison approaches					
Pairwise comparison	change in values reconceptualization	can be time-consuming; burden may be mitigated by using multi-media software	well-established; reference point and context can influence value assigned	well-established	strong empirical background
Card sorting	change in values reconceptualization	requires cards to accompany self-report questionnaire; can be confusing for cognitively-impaired patients; potentially time-consuming	forced distribution can result in increased random error	long-history of use in ipsative measurement supports its construct validity	yes

Table continues

Table 6.1. *(Continued)*

Method	Aspect(s) of response shift measured	Feasibility	Reliability established?	Validity established?	Empirical data available?
Design approaches					
Then-Test	change in internal standards reconceptualization inferred	easily accommodates existing measures and brief Then-Test can be constructed using pilot data; potentially time-consuming if one uses entire scale rather than item subsets with Then Test instructions	would be similar to reliability of measure being adapted	yes, in educational research; there is some question about its being confounded with recall bias	numerous studies have successfully applied the method to educational research; applications to QOL in progress
Ideal scale approach	change in internal standards change in values reconceptualization	time-consuming because it doubles the self-report questionnaires collected	ceiling effects can be mitigated by specifying anchors	yes, in organizational change; must clarify meaning of 'ideal' to minimize ambiguity for QOL research	used in studies of organizational change
Statistical approaches					
Covariance/factor analysis	change in internal standards reconceptualization	no additional measures required; can require large samples unless informal method used; cannot address the nature of the reconceptualization	may suffer from problems of unreliable factor structure if appropriate subject-to-variable ratio not maintained; informal analyses may be useful	convergent validity not established	yes; support not using such approaches without triangulating other approaches

Growth curve analysis	infers existence of response shift, rather than directly assessing change in internal standards, changes in values or reconceptualization	available, parsimonious, handles missing data well; requires comparison group and additional data to assess response shift	NR	NR	yes; increasingly used in longitudinal social science research
Qualitative methods					
Idiographic assessment of personal goals	change in values reconceptualization	can be time-consuming and resource-intensive	can suffer from low reliability	NA	yes; increasingly used in longitudinal social science research

Note. NA = not currently available. NR = not relevant. Psychometric criteria are not relevant for growth curve and extended Q-TWiST methods.

Individualized Methods

General description. This family of methods attempts to make the concerns of the individual central to defining and measuring relevant QOL domains for the individual. All of these methods require integrating individual patient feedback in defining QOL by identifying the relevant domains, anchors and importance weights which are used to generate QOL outcome scores (Jambon & Johnson, 1997). Some of these methods require in-person interviews, whereas others rely on paper-and-pencil measures to elicit such idiographic data. There are numerous methods of this type (Allison et al., 1997; Jambon & Johnson, 1997). Rather than describing all of the methods within this family, three examples will be described. The interested reader is referred to primary sources to learn more about other techniques, such as the Patient Generated Index (Ruta et al., 1994); the Problem Elicitation Technique (Bakker et al., 1995) and the Subjective Domains of QOL Measure (Bar-On & Amir, 1993; Amir et al., 1994).

Example 1: the Repertory Grid Technique. The Repertory Grid Technique (Thunedborg et al., 1993) asks patients to define those aspects of life that are important to their health, well-being and functioning. For example, patients might be asked to compare their perception of or reaction to real or imaginary persons in different life situations. This method assumes that QOL is relational and thus determined by discrepancies between their current self on the one hand and their past abilities, future aspirations and peers' current functioning on the other.

Example 2: Cantril's Ladder. Cantril's Ladder (Cantril, 1966) elicits respondents to rate their current life satisfaction on a ladder that ranges from 0 to 10, where 0 reflects worst imaginable life satisfaction and 10 reflects best imaginable life satisfaction. Respondents are first asked to describe these two anchors and then to rate their current life satisfaction on this ideographically-anchored continuum.

Example 3: the Schedule for the Evaluation of Individual Quality of Life (SEIQoL). The Schedule for the Evaluation of Individual Quality of Life (SEIQoL) (O'Boyle et al., 1992; Browne et al., 1994; O'Boyle, 1994) requires that patients nominate the five most relevant domains to their QOL. They then assess their current status within each domain using a visual analogue scale with anchors ranging from 'best possible' to 'worst possible.' Judgement analysis is used to rank the relative importance of each domain, based on patient ratings of 30 hypothetical QOL scenarios for the five referenced domains. The SEIQoL generates an overall index that summarizes satisfaction with and relative importance of each domain.

Assessing response shift with individualized methods. Although not the original intent of these measures, they can be adapted to measure different aspects of response shift using the following general method. First, one can repeat the described exercises at subsequent assessment points and compare the described anchors (Cantril's Ladder) and/or domains (the Repertory Grid and the SEIQoL). With respect to the anchors, the comparison might begin by asking patients to describe the relevant anchors both at time 1 (T1) and time 2 (T2). At T2 patients could be asked to place their T1 anchors within the T2-anchored continuum. This approach is a way of evaluating change in internal standards by making explicit patients' change in anchors over time and the relationship between the anchors over time. Additionally, the changing content of the anchors reflects a reconceptualization of the target construct. With respect to the domains, the changing context of the domains is indicative of two kinds of changes. First, a change in values would be suggested by changes in the order of the domains. Second, a change in conceptualization would be suggested by changes in the content of the domains.

Evaluation. These approaches are feasible albeit labor intensive as they require in-person, semi-structured interviews and require that one provide feedback using baseline data. It is possible that multimedia computer-assisted presentations may be adapted to facilitate these methods (cf. Lenert et al., 1997; Soetikno et al., 1997). Their psychometric characteristics (i.e. reliability and validity) are expected to be comparable to the original methods, so investigators would be encouraged to utilize outcome measures with strong psychometric properties. Because some of these methods use single-item measures which have low reliability, those that sample multiple domains in addition to an overall assessment of QOL are preferred. These methods would assess concomitantly at least two of the three aspects of response shift, i.e. change in internal standards, reconceptualization, change in values. Future investigations are needed to develop feasible, reproducible ways of summarizing change in internal standards as well as for scoring the content analysis of the qualitative data on reconceptualization or change in values. Since these methods have not yet been applied to assess response shift, there are no empirical data available at this time.

Preference-based Methods

General description. These methods assess the importance and value a patient explicitly places on a health state or quality-of-life dimension (Ditto et al., 1996). For example, patients are asked to rate the value of a particular health state using a visual analogue scale (e.g. a feeling thermometer), where 1 reflects perfect health and 0 refers to death. Other methods ask patients to make explicit exchanges to reveal their values. For example, in the time trade-off approach (Torrance, 1986), patients are asked to make choices between longevity and living in a better state of health. As an exhaustive review is beyond the scope of the present work, one example of a preference-based method will be provided which may integrate response shift into treatment evaluations and one example of how preferences or utilities might be used to assess response shift.

Example 1: the Extended Q-TWiST method. The Extended Q-TWiST method (Schwartz et al., 1995a, 1995b) is a special case of any of a number of techniques which use a quality adjusted life year (QALY) model based on individual patient-generated utilities at each point in time. In contrast to other preference-based approaches where patient importance ratings are elicited at one point in time, an Extended Q-TWiST requires collecting patient importance ratings over time for each QOL domain assessed and collecting data on the social cost impact (e.g. work disability, institutionalization) of a given disease or treatment. A weighted assessment score is computed which represents severity of symptoms for each dimension measured, weighted by its patient-derived preference value at each data collection time point. This score is then used to compute (QALYs), which summarize the amount of healthy or quality time an individual patient enjoys over the course of follow-up.

Assessing response shift with the Extended Q-TWiST. By integrating preference values at each time point, the Extended Q-TWiST incorporates changes in values. Consequently, changes in importance ratings or preference assessments would assess response shift and treatment evaluations which implement an Extended Q-TWiST analysis would implicitly integrate response shift effects with respect to changes in values.

Evaluation of the Extended Q-TWiST method. This method provides a promising and feasible avenue for integrating response shift into treatment evaluation. There are data available which suggest that preference weights fluctuate over the course of treatment, implying that the method may be sensitive to response shift resulting from changes in values (e.g. Schwartz et al., 1997). These changes may integrate changing tolerance to treatment costs and benefits. This method is limited by the potential patient burden involved in collecting preferences or utilities at each point in time. Rather than being an assessment tool, the Extended Q-TWiST provides a way of analyzing QOL and preference data. Consequently, its reliability and validity are contingent upon the QOL and clinical measures which are integrated in the analysis.

Example 2: the Preference Mapping method. One method which is currently being developed by Schwartz and colleagues attempts to use preferences or utilities collected over time to estimate changes in values. This Preference Mapping method requires collecting preference or utility data over time on several invariant health states, as well as on the patient's own health state. Additionally, criterion data on the patients' objective level of function needs to be collected. The invariant health states should describe states that are proximal to the patient's own health state. These invariant health states can be defined based on descriptions which combine levels of functioning as measured by standardized scales (see Sugar et al., 1998). Shifts in the patients' value function for these health states would then be mapped or plotted over time. Non-linear models would examine how patients' values for health states change as a function of changes in their own health over time.

Assessing response shift with the Preference Mapping method. Changes in values would be reflected by a shift in patient preference values for their own state. Values for those states that are proximal to their own may also change. If the patient's objective function had not changed over time, then one would expect a linear function with a slope of zero. If the patient's objective function had changed, then the patient would have undergone a loss or gain in health which would influence his/her value function. If no response shift in values had occurred, then one would predict a linear function with a non-zero slope. If a response shift in values had occurred, however, then one would predict a non-linear relationship between the health state ratings (i.e. preference values or utilities) at the two time points.[1]

Non-linear models, such as those derived from hysteretic models, will be useful for assessing response shift using preference data collected over time. A hysteretic model lends itself to quantifying response shift by describing time-dependent changes in path from one reference point to another using first or second order differential equations (Mayergoyz, 1991).[2]

Evaluation of the Preference Mapping method. This method requires collecting preference data for several health states at each data collection time point and thus may be time-consuming. Complex statistical techniques are required to implement this approach to assessing response shift, a consideration which may be a disadvantage. This difficulty can be minimized once computer software has been developed to do Preference Mapping data collection (i.e. utility elicitation) and analysis for the end user. The Preference Mapping method is currently under development and will require development of specific non-linear models to measure changes in values. At present, its sensitivity to response shift is unknown and is a promising area for future research.

---

[1]The specific predictions for the slope and non-linearity of the changes from this Preference Mapping method are based upon Prospect Theory (Kahneman and Tversky, 1979). Prospect Theory predicts that values are treated as a function of two arguments: the asset position that serves as the reference point, and the magnitude of the change from that reference point. The value function can be characterized as S-shaped, with health state losses resulting in a steep overestimate of the value of that worsened state and significant health state gains leading to a slight underestimate of the value of that improved state.

[2]Hysteresis refers to the idea that we cannot understand or explain present outcomes without reference to the past. That is, one returns from a health state change using a different path (i.e. set of values) than how one got there, and one returns to a 'perturbed' (i.e. new) reference point. This concept has been extensively developed by economists (Setterfield, 1997) and pharmacokineticists (Sheiner, 1985) in the past decade and would appear to have applications to the field of QOL research. Hysteresis equations describe non-reversible loops of history dependence, such that extreme rather than moderate experiences are postulated to influence future behavior (Cross, 1993). Defining these extreme values is done by threshold estimation (Freidlin and Pfeiffer, 1998), a step that would be particularly relevant to response shift research inasmuch as it enables one to identify what level of health state change constitutes a 'catalyst.'

Successive Comparison Approaches

General description. This family of methods involves making a series of judgements about the ordering or ranking of objects along a psychological or physical continuum. This ordering could be done by presenting the objects in all possible pairs and asking the individuals to judge which member of the pair was highest on the parameter of interest. These comparisons of relative importance would be done over time.

Example 1: pairwise comparisons. This well-established approach described by Edwards (1957) could be applied to the context of assessing response shift as follows. Patients could be asked to rate the importance of a series of domains by successively comparing two sets of domains with each other at least twice over time. The relative importance over time would reflect response shift in terms of changes in values. If the patient were allowed to select the domains for which the pairwise comparison would be done, then this method would also reflect reconceptualization.

Evaluation of pairwise comparison. The advantage of the pairwise comparison method is that the method itself is well-established and reliable. The disadvantage, however, is that the process can be somewhat burdensome as it results in a large number of potential combinations which can be time-consuming for data collection. For example, 10 objects would require 45 pairs to be analyzed (i.e. number of pairs = (number of objects) * (number of objects − 1)/2). Additionally, the reliability of the pairwise comparison method may be compromised by the fact that framing or context may result in different choices or ranking (Kahneman & Tversky, 1979), independent of a true response shift.

Example 2: the card sort approach. In this approach, patients are given a sorting sheet which forces distinct importance rankings for each QOL domain in question (Schwartz, 1996) (Fig. 6.1). This approach is similar to a Q-Sort methodology (Stephenson, 1953) which attempted to allow investigators to examine correlations between different conditions for the same person (Wittenborn, 1961). Like the pairwise comparison technique, the Card Sort approach might be used to assess changes in values. If patients can choose their own domains, then this method can reflect reconceptualization.

Evaluation of card sort methods. The card sort method has a well-established foundation in ipsative measurement (Stephenson, 1953; Wittenborn, 1961). Additionally, a recent investigation of a card sort method to evaluate coping variability with life stressors suggested that such methods may be best analyzed using non-linear dynamical analysis (Schwartz et al., 1998). The card sort method requires that the investigator send along with the self-report questionnaire a special set of cards containing the QOL domains of interest, a disadvantage since the cards may be misplaced by patients. A second disadvantage is that the process can be con-

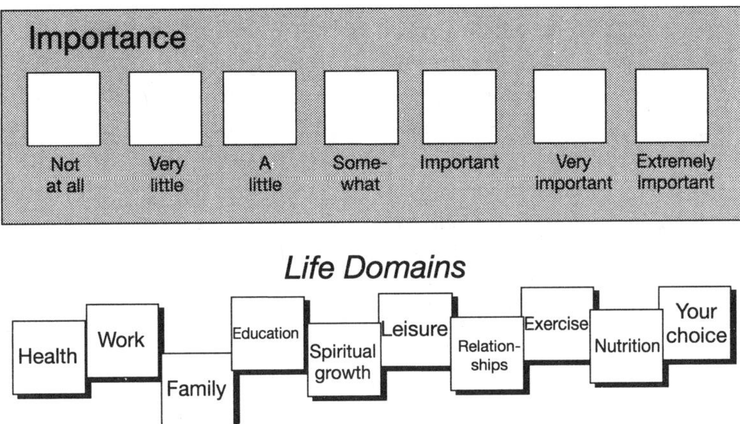

Figure 6.1. A card sort game to assess values. The card sort approach forces distinct importance rankings for each QOL domain. Changes in ranking over time would reflect response shifts in values and the conceptualization of QOL.

fusing for cognitively-impaired patients. Finally, the method can be time-consuming.

Design Approaches

General description. This family of methods confronts the challenge of assessing response shift by imposing study design changes which are intended to elucidate one or more aspects of response shift.

Example 1: the Then Test. Perhaps the best established approach is the retrospective-pretest design, which includes a Then Test as a way of evaluating changes in internal standards. Originating in the discipline of educational training interventions, this method requires that at the posttest, patients are asked to fill out the self-report measure in reference to how they perceive themselves to have been prior to the intervention (Then Test). Thus, at the Then Test subjects are asked to provide a renewed judgement about their pre-treatment level of functioning.

Assessing response shift with the Then Test. The conventional posttest and Then Test measures are presumed to be completed with the same internal standard of measurement since they are collected at the same time. Consequently, comparison of posttest and Then Test scores would eliminate treatment-induced response-shift effects and provide an unconfounded indication of the treatment effect. The comparison of the mean pretest and Then Test scores would reflect an estimate of the amount and direction of response-shift effects (see Sprangers et al., 1999, for empirical example of this approach). The Then Test can be implemented on entire measures or on selected items. One should select items where response shift would be expected to occur (e.g. subjective outcomes). For validation purposes, one might also want to include items where response shift is less likely to occur (e.g. objective outcomes). Within this conceptual selection, one can choose items which yield adequate reliability and validity. For example, one might choose items which lower the scale's alpha reliability when deleted (i.e., lower deleted alpha) and which have a relatively high correlation with the scale's or subscale's total score. This psychometrically-driven item selection would minimize the patient burden while ensuring that the better items within a given subscale were included as Then Test items.

Evaluation of the Then Test approach. Although this method originated in education evaluation research, its application to health-related QOL research is relatively recent and limited (cf. Sprangers & van Dam, 1994; Sprangers, 1996). Besides reflecting changes in internal standards, this method infers reconceptualization since a response scale which is expanded or contracted based upon experience may necessarily relate to changes in conceptualization (see Section Discussion). The majority of studies which included a Then Test in the design were performed in the area of educational research. These studies revealed changes in the expected direction or, alternatively, revealed larger intervention effects than those revealed by the conventional pretest–posttest design (e.g. Howard & Dailey, 1979; Howard et al., 1979b, 1979c; Hoogstraten, 1982, 1985; Sprangers, 1988, 1989; Sprangers & Hoogstraten, 1987, 1989; Levinson et al., 1990; Skeff et al., 1992; Sprangers et al., 1999). The Then Test was also found to be more strongly associated with objective criteria of change (Howard et al., 1979a; Bray & Howard, 1980; Howard et al., 1981; Stieglitz, 1990; Skeff et al., 1992), suggesting that this approach may be a more accurate and sensitive assessment of respondent's perspective on personal change. There is some question about its being confounded with recall bias. Response shift effects revealed by this method, however, have been found to be more prevalent for subjective rather than objective outcomes, suggesting that the Then Test is measuring something distinct from recall bias (Schwartz & Lee, 1998). The use of the Then Test for assessing response shift in symptoms may be better applied to symptoms which are prevalent at baseline (Sprangers et al., 1999). One disadvantage of this method is the need to include extra measures. Investigators interested in using this approach should be careful to apply it to measures with strong psychometric properties, since the Then Test will have similar reliability to that of the measure being adapted. It should be noted that the Then Test approach does not mitigate the need for baseline assessment. Future research should address the optimal time interval for accurate Then Test measurement and should test the viability of alternative explanations (e.g. social desirability, cognitive dissonance) than response shift for explaining variance in Then Test scores.

Example 2: the ideal scale approach. With its roots in organizational change research, the ideal scale approach was originally designed for situations where respondents were asked about their opinions of others (e.g. leader behavior; Zmud & Armenakis, 1978; Armenakis & Zmud, 1979). However, this design approach can be easily adapted to refer to self-reported QOL. The logic of employing an ideal scale was to obtain a standard of measurement or criterion to enable detection of changes in internal standards (Armenakis, 1988). Respondents are asked to complete a questionnaire twice: first in reference to their actual status (e.g. how they perceive their current QOL) and second to their ideal status (e.g. how they would like their QOL to be). These two questionnaires are administered at different points in time. Changes in internal standards would be captured by significant changes in ideal scores over time. If changes in internal standards have thus been detected, the difference scores between the ideal and the actual scales at each point in time would be used to assess unconfounded (behavioral) change.

Assessing response shift with the ideal scale approach. While the method is aimed at detecting changes in internal standards, it is conceivable that this method might also be useful in detecting changes in values and conceptualization. For example, respondents might be asked to indicate the relative importance of QOL domains currently and ideally. Changes in the 'ideal' hierarchy of QOL domains would thus be indicative of value changes. Relatedly, patients could be asked to define their 'ideal' QOL. Changes over time in such definitions would reflect reconceptualization.

Evaluation of the ideal scale approach. While the original approach is feasible, it increases patient burden by doubling the questionnaires at each time point. The psychometric characteristics (i.e. reliability and validity) of the 'ideal' QOL questionnaire in comparison to the questionnaire assessing actual QOL may be limited due to restriction of range that may result from ceiling effects (Terborg et al., 1980, 1982; Schmitt et al., 1984). Thus, this approach may be useful but will require selecting questionnaires that are less susceptible to ceiling effects. To circumvent ceiling effects, respondents may be asked about their ambitions (Calman, 1984), expectations or potential achievements (Powell, 1987), rather than about their ideal QOL. Whatever anchor is being used, it needs to be clearly defined and this definition should be held constant across time in order to detect changes in internal standards. Two laboratory studies in the field of organizational change (Buckley & Armenakis, 1987; Granier et al., 1991) indicated that the ideal scale approach was able to detect clearly changes in internal standards and was found to be unaffected by ceiling effects. An additional concern with this approach is that 'ideal' needs to be defined. For example, it may refer to what a person would like, expects, or strives for. While this design approach is aimed at assessing changes in internal standards, it is conceivable that over time, the concept 'ideal' may change from 'what might ideally happen' to a more realistic 'what can reasonably be expected' (see also Terborg et al., 1982). In this sense, the method may not sufficiently distinguish changes in internal standards from changes in conceptualization. This design approach has not yet been applied to QOL research.

Statistical Approaches

General description. This family of approaches would evaluate longitudinal data for statistical trends which suggest an underlying response shift. We will present only two examples of such statistical approaches, although it is likely that there are a number of other methods which could be described.

Example 1: covariance/factor analysis. Researchers in the area of organizational change have suggested a range of statistical approaches to detect reconceptualization. Each approach evaluates longitudinal data for dissimilarities in factor structure. They differ in the way they subsequently analyze and compare these sets of responses. The Transformation Method (Golembiewski et al., 1976) is aimed at detecting changes in the factor structure of the two assessments. Different factor structures are deemed indicative of reconceptualization. A factor-by-factor comparison is purported to reveal which aspect of the target construct may have been reconceptualized. However, it is unclear at which level of dissimilarity between the factor solutions (pattern and/or magnitude) the conclusion of reconceptualization is warranted. The advantage of the Coefficients of Congruence Method (Armenakis et al., 1977; Bedeian et al., 1988), which also examines the similarity of factor structures, is that it provides a test for statistical significance of the congruence coefficients (Korth & Tucker, 1975). Relatedly, Schmitt (1982) proposed the Analysis of Covariance Structures using LISREL (Jöreskog & Sörbom, 1981). In addition to the inspection of factor structures, Schmitt recommends testing for the homogeneity of the variance–covariance structures. This LISREL approach is meant to reveal reconceptualization. The Transformation Method (Golembiewski et al., 1976) and the Analysis of Covariance Structures (Schmitt, 1982; Schmitt et al., 1984) are also proposed to identify change in internal standards. However, the heuristic guidelines provided may be challenged for their general and imprecise nature (Armenakis, 1988).

Evaluation of the covariance/factor analysis. These statistical approaches have the advantage that no extra measures are required, in contrast to the majority of the other methods described in this paper. However, these approaches require relatively large sample sizes which may limit their feasibility. For example, if an appropriate subject-to-variable ratio is not maintained, covariance/factor analytic methods may suggest factor structures which are unreliable due to random error. This problem might be mitigated by using the factor structure output less formally. For example, one might look at the relative importance of component domains by looking at the proportion of the total variance explained by one item or subscale within a factor (cf. Schwartz et al., 1997). One might then examine whether relative importance changes over time. Other aspects which set limits to their usefulness (and may compromise their reliability and validity) are the number of assumptions and requirements that may be violated. For example, the Coefficients of Congruence Method requires that the factor structures being compared must contain a similar number of factors. Further, while these statistical approaches are based on the administration of similar items over time, one may argue their suitability to assess reconceptualization. Major changes in the conceptualization of the target construct are not likely to be captured by simply using the original questionnaire items. Even if these methods were capable of unequivocally identifying reconceptualization, they would not reveal the nature of this change (Norman & Parker, 1996). Two studies assessing the convergent validity of these methods in assessing reconceptualization by using a common data set (Armenakis et al., 1982; Schmitt et al., 1984), showed that the convergent validity among the three methods is questionable. Additionally, there is no empirical evidence of the methods' convergent validity in detecting change in internal standards. Finally, it should be noted that the statistical approaches were originally designed to assess reconceptualization and further 'adapted' to capture change in internal standards. This is never explicitly stated but it is implicated in the way they are described and in their respective weaknesses. The lack of clear guidelines to distinguish reconceptualization from change in internal standards led Armenakis (1988) to wonder whether these methods accurately detect reconceptualization and change in internal standards and to call for further investigations into these methods. Given the many drawbacks of these statistical techniques, we would recommend supplementing them with at least one of the other methods described in this paper (e.g. individualized techniques, design approaches) (see also Norman & Parker, 1996).

Example 2: growth curve analysis. This relatively new technique computes individual slopes to assess change over time on the dependent variable of interest (Rogosa et al., 1982; Willett et al., 1991; Francis et al., 1992).[3] In contrast to more conventional linear models, which generally focus on group means or proportions, growth curve models focus on the individual growth trajectories of each person (or any given individual unit of interest). The technique is quite flexible and a wide variety of problems that have plagued traditional repeated measures models can be addressed in a very efficient and illuminating manner (e.g. heterogeneity of variance, autocorrelation, etc., see for example, Littel et al., 1996). Of particular note is that growth curve models also allow the investigator to explore variables

[3]With origins in earlier work on time series analysis (e.g. Elston & Grizzle, 1962) and mixed or variance components models (e.g. Cochran & Cox, 1957), growth curve models are also closely related to more recent approaches, such as random effect models (Laird & Ware, 1982), empirical Bayes estimation (Lindley & Smith, 1972), hierarchical linear or multilevel models (Bryk & Raudenbush, 1987).

that might influence both the overall level (intercept) and the trajectory (slope) of individual change (Bryk & Raudenbush, 1987). Moreover, recent advances have also made it possible to formally assess the relation between two or more curves (Willett & Sayer, 1996).

Assessing response shift with growth curve analysis. Growth curve modeling can be useful for inferring response shift in existing data, but it is not likely to lead to direct estimates of any of the three aspects of response shift. For example, comparing the functional form of the growth in subjective and objective indices of QOL might reveal a disengagement of the two and may indicate that response shift is occurring (cf. Schwartz, 1999). This inference assumes that as people get sicker, they will also become more distressed. If patients with a progressive disability do not report increased distress, one might infer that their reference point for distress is changing. Growth curve analysis might be useful as a first step in primary or secondary analysis to determine whether response shift is likely to have occurred.

Evaluation of growth curve analysis. This statistical approach represents a promising direction for exploring patterns of change in longitudinal QOL data and inferring the existence of response shift. It is a feasible method of analyzing data which is available in the more commonly-used statistical software for the social sciences. Growth curve modeling is also more sensitive to change, accommodates missing data well, and is more parsimonious than repeated measures ANOVA (Speer and Greenbaum, 1995; Nich & Carroll, 1997). This method does not measure the different aspects of response shift directly, however, so one would still need to collect data on response shift directly. Further, including comparison groups (e.g. healthy versus sick; progressive versus stable patients) would be necessary to infer that the disengagement of subjective and objective indices might indeed imply response shift.

Overall evaluation of statistical methods. An inherent feature of statistical methods is that they are model-based, which has two substantial advantages. First, they force the researcher to think about the system behind the response shift. Second, they allow one to test several hypotheses about response shift and their aspects. The disadvantage is that they may not allow one to derive a response shift score which could be used and interpreted.

Qualitative Methods

General description. Qualitative approaches for evaluating response shift would involve developing semi-structured interviews which are aimed at probing respondents so that they can delineate their experience. Examples of such approaches would include focus groups or semi-structured interviews. We will describe one example of such qualitative approaches, although it should be noted that the individualized approaches also contain qualitative aspects.

An example: the Idiographic Assessment of Personal Goals. Rapkin and Fischer (1992) and Rapkin et al. (1994) have developed a two-part structured interview to investigate respondents' goals as well as their self-evaluation of these goals. Probes are used to elicit types of goals using open-ended questions such as "What things would you like to achieve or accomplish?" and "What things do you want to avoid or prevent from happening?" In the second part of the interview, respondents are asked to rate their goals on a series of dimensions, such as level of effort needed to pursue the goal, time frame, commitment required, etc. The first part of this approach is then amenable to content analysis, whereas the latter results in scores more commonly used in quantitative social science.

Assessing response shift with the Idiographic Assessment of Personal Goals. Response shift would be evident in the change in goal content from one interview to the next and would be apparent based on the content analysis. Change in goal content would reflect reconceptualization, while change in values would be reflected by a reordering of the goal priorities.

Evaluation of the Idiographic Assessment of Personal Goals. Qualitative methods can yield rich data and present promising alternatives for hypothesis generation and for gaining a richer understanding of a phenomenon (cf. Sprangers et al., 1999; Schwartz & Sendor, 1999). Finally, the questions can be specified so that one aspect of response shift is explored in some depth, thereby providing a foundation for further conceptual distinction between the three aspects of response shift. The disadvantages of qualitative methods are that they can be time-consuming to implement and require ample resources for data extraction and analysis. Further, their open-ended format can result in relatively low reliability within a respondent's answers at two time points (Rapkin, personal communication, November 7, 1997). Finally these methods, like numerous other self-report measures, rely on respondents' introspection about and awareness of the phenomenon being measured. Response shift may have significant pre-cognitive components which are not yet within the purview of respondents' awareness. This awareness can also be influenced by how the questions are phrased and the information sought. Qualitative methods might be more susceptible to reactivity and to demand characteristics than paper-and-pencil self-report measures, so the questions should be selected and implemented with care.

Discussion

We have discussed a number of methods which could be adapted or further developed to investigate response shift. The more established methods (e.g. those originating from educational or organizational change) have been discussed more critically than the relatively new methods because empirical evidence is available on the former to highlight their drawbacks. Consequently, the discussion of the respective methods has been necessarily unbalanced. Because very few methods have been designed specifically to assess response shift and empirical data are available for only a few measures in areas other than QOL, there is a strong need to conduct further research on these methods. It should be noted that a number of the methods require that people define QOL domains or goals (i.e. ipsative). Thus, one might also distinguish the methods from one another in terms of whether they are ipsative or normative.

It is apparent that one of the greatest challenges facing this area of research is that the majority of the available measures operationalize more than one aspect of response shift (see Table 6.1). It may be the case that these aspects of response shift are ineluctably intertwined and that respecting this inter-connection between internal standards, values and conceptualization may be a crucial step to allowing this phenomenon to elucidate heretofore unexplained paradoxes in health-related QOL research. For example, response shift may be a useful construct in investigating the uniformly high levels of patient satisfaction reported in various surveys (Carr-Hill, 1992), as patients change their perceptions and values over the course of care (Avis et al., 1997).

This inter-connection may also reflect a hierarchical nature. For example, researchers in the field of alpha, beta and gamma change have adopted the following hierarchy: first, gamma change needs to be ruled out before beta change can be detected and then beta change needs to be ruled out before alpha change can be identified. This approach makes sense since change in internal standards will have lost its meaning if the construct itself is dissimilar at two time points. Conversely, it is difficult to imagine that change in internal standards might occur without affecting the meaning of the construct. If the response scale (Fig. 6.2a) is expanded (or contracted) based on experience (Fig. 6.2b), then the anchors (and the intervals) have different meaning (Fig. 6.2c). For example, the individualized methods assume that a change over time in anchor descriptions

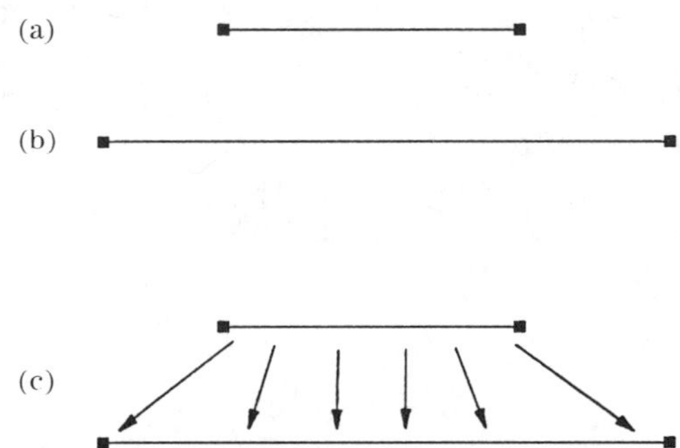

Figure 6.2. Change in internal standards may be ineluctably related to reconceptualization. If the response scale (a) is expanded (or contracted) based on experience (b), then the anchors (and the intervals) have different meaning (c).

(a)

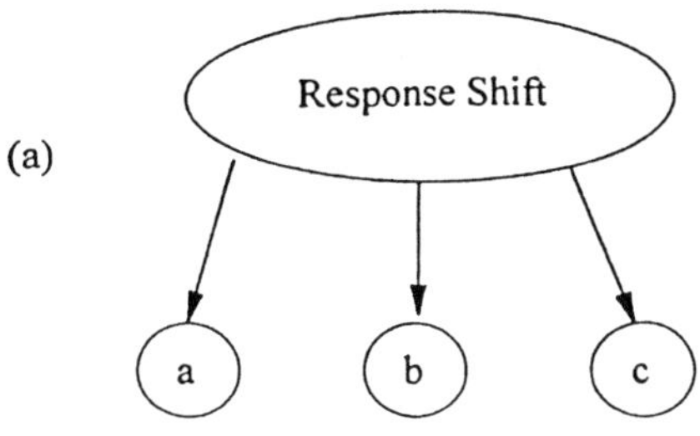

(b)

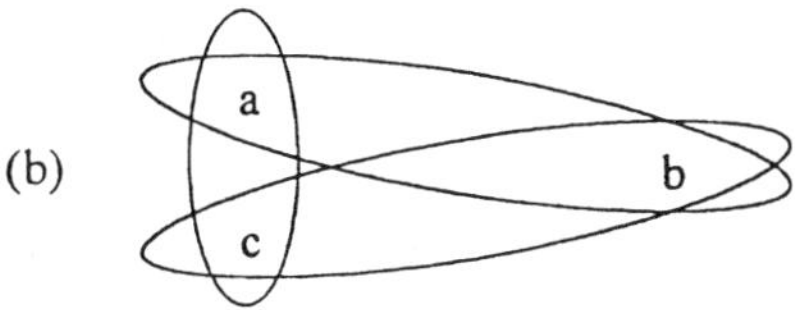

Figure 6.3. Rather than assuming that response shift is a latent variable with distinct operationalizations (a), a better approach might be to triangulate assessment (b) so that algebraic formulae be used to yield balanced scores reflecting each aspect of response shift.

reflects change in internal standards. It is possible, however, that this change might also reflect reconceptualization. Thus, clearly distinguishing the three aspects of response shift may be a desired convenience for researchers more than a true reflection of the phenomenon.

Rather than assuming that response shift is a latent variable with distinct operationalizations (Fig. 6.3a), a better approach might be to develop algebraic formulae for converting triangulated measures into balanced scores reflecting each aspect of response shift (Fig. 6.3b). It may be the case that the components of response shift can only reflect the construct when measured in pairs. For example, change in internal standards may only reflect response shift when it is coincident with changes in values or changes in conceptualization. Change in internal standards by itself might only reflect measurement error. Thus, if one collected data using several measures which operationalize in conjunction aspects a and b; a and c; and b and c, for example:

$$\text{Response Shift}_{\text{operationalization}} = u_{ab} + v_{bc} + w_{ac}.$$

One might solve for a (i.e. change in internal standards), b (i.e. reconceptualization) and c (i.e. change in values) using the following formulae:

$$a = \frac{u + w}{u_{ab} + v_{bc} + w_{ac}};$$

$$b = \frac{u + v}{u_{ab} + v_{bc} + w_{ac}};$$

$$c = \frac{v + w}{u_{ab} + v_{bc} + w_{ac}}$$

where u refers to the number of measures which operationalize aspects a and b of response shift; v refers to the number of measures which operationalize aspects b and c of response shift; and w refers to the number of measures which operationalize aspects a and c of response shift. To get a balanced portrayal of aspects a, b and c, one would simply sum the numbers resulting from the above algebraic formulae (i.e. response shift = $a + b + c$). This algebraic approach merits some development although it faces a significant challenge not unknown to QOL researchers, that of translating different questionnaires to a comparable metric despite differences in content, metric and scope.

Triangulating methods would thus be a useful direction for future research. By combining the information available using more than one method, one might also reveal relevant information which can be elucidated by other methods. For example, collecting Then Test data might evaluate how patients changed their internal standards or reconceptualized QOL with respect to a referent time point. Combining this information with the Preference Mapping approach and growth curve analysis might yield testable models for understanding how these changes in standards and conceptualizations relate to changes in values, and how all three aspects of response shift contribute to different trajectories in perceived QOL.

There are a small number of studies which have triangulated different techniques in evaluating response shift. For example, comparisons have been made between design and statistical approaches. Schmitt et al. (1984) compared their Analysis of Covariance Structure approach with the Ideal Scale and the Then Test design approaches in detecting change in internal standards. The LISREL and the Then Test approaches concurred. Randolph and Elloy (1989) have compared the Coefficients of Congruence Method and the Then Test approach in detecting reconceptualization. There was some consistency between the two techniques. These types of studies are promising and merit further exploration.

A final issue which should be further explored is that the phenomenon may not always be within the individual's awareness. If the phenomenon is pre-cognitive, then methods for evaluating response shift might focus more on *demonstrating* changes in internal standards, values and conceptualization rather than asking respondents to report on these aspects directly.

This paper has discussed a variety of existing and new methods that can be used for assessing response shift phenomenon. It thus attempts to facilitate the operationalization of one component of the theoretical model proposed by Sprangers and Schwartz (1999). It should be noted, however, that our current level of understanding of this phenomenon is limited. Consequently, we have decided to impose few restrictions on the specificity of these methods in evaluating one or another aspect of response shift. Further, some of the distinctions we made between methods may be more apparent than real (e.g. overlap between individualized and qualitative methods). Future research should validate the described measures in terms of criterion and content validity and should investigate the described methods for potential threats to their internal validity.

Despite the limitations in our current understanding of this phenomenon, there are some guidelines which may be useful for investigators interested in implementing response shift research. The primary guideline would be to include criterion measures of change in response shift study designs so that investigators can distinguish objective change from changes in internal standards, values and conceptualization. Second, triangulating alternative methods should be standard in response shift studies, both to reveal all the components of response shift as well as to validate the various methods. Third, strong theory-driven hypotheses are required for rigorous development of the construct. It would thus be wise to think about the system behind response shift and to aim to be model-based in using both statistical and non-statistical methods. Including comparison groups in a study would be helpful for testing hypotheses, for delineating the catalysts of response shift, and for examining the adaptive and maladaptive implications of response shift. For those researchers who are interested in further developing the construct, they might consider testing the Sprangers and Schwartz (1999) theoretical model of response shift. Fourth, response shift studies should be implemented in a variety of settings and contexts (e.g. pharmaceutical studies, disease-management evaluations, psychosocial intervention studies, patient satisfaction studies) so that its importance and implications can be delineated. Finally, it is important that zealous investigators continue to entertain the possibility that factors other than response shift may play a role in study outcomes. It is the hope that enumerating possible tools using existing and new methods will make it easier for other researchers in diverse fields to collaborate in the development of this emerging construct.

References

Allison, P. J., Locker, D., & Feine, J. S. (1997). Quality of life: A dynamic construct. *Social Science and Medicine*, *45*, 221–230.

Amir, M., Bar-On, D., & Cristal, N. (1994). Quality of life in hypertensives and normotensives in Israel: Introducing a self-structured subjective measure. In J. Orley & W. Kuyken (Eds.), *Quality of life assessment: International perspectives*. (pp. 177–184). Berlin: Springer-Verlag.

Armenakis, A. A. (1988). A review of research on the change typology. *Research in Organizational Change and Development*, *2*, 163–194.

Armenakis, A., Feild, H., & Wilmoth, J. (1977). An algorithm for assessing factor structure congruence. *Educational and Psychological Measurement*, *37*, 213–214.

Armenakis, A., Randolph, W., & Bedeian, A. (1982, March 17–22). A comparison of two methods for evaluating the similarity of factor analysis solutions. In *Proceedings of the Southwest Academy of Management Meeting* (pp. 138–142). Dallas, TX.

Armenakis, A. A., & Zmud, R. (1979). Interpreting the measurement of change in organizational research. *Personnel Psychology*, *32*, 709–723.

Avis, M., Bond, M., & Arthur, A. (1997). Questioning patient satisfaction: An empirical investigation in two outpatient clinics. *Social Science and Medicine*, *44*, 85–92.

Bakker, C., van der Linden, S., van Santen-Hoeufft, M., Bolwijn, P., & Hidding, A. (1995). Problem elicitation to assess patient priorities in ankyloring spondylitis and fibromyalgia. *Journal of Rheumatology*, *22*, 1304–1310.

Bar-On, D., & Amir, M. (1993). Re-examining quality of life of hypertensives: A new self-structured measure. *American Journal of Hypertension, 6*, 62S–66S.

Bedeian, A., Armenakis, A., & Randolph, W. (1988). The significance of congruence coefficients: A comment and statistical test. *Journal of Management, 14*, 559–566.

Bray, J. H., & Howard, G. S. (1980). Methodological considerations in the evaluation of a teacher-training program. *Journal of Educational Psychology, 72*, 62–70.

Browne, J. P., O'Boyle, C. A., McGee, H. M., Joyce, C. R. B., McDonald, N. J., O'Malley, K., & Hiltbrunner, B. (1994). Individual quality of life in the healthy elderly. *Quality of Life Research, 3*, 235–244.

Bryk, A. S., & Raudenbush, S. W. (1987). Application of hierarchical linear models to assessing change. *Psychological Bulletin, 101*(1), 147–158.

Buckley, M., & Armenakis, A. A. (1987). Detecting scale recalibration in survey research: A laboratory investigation. *Group and Organization Studies, 12*, 464–481.

Calman, K. C. (1984). Quality of life in cancer patients: An hypothesis. *Journal of Medical Ethics, 10*, 124–127.

Cantril, H. (1966). *The pattern of human concerns*. New Brunswick, NJ: Rutgers University Press.

Carr-Hill, R. (1992). The measurement of patient satisfaction. *Journal of Public Health Medicine, 14*, 236–249.

Cochran, W. G., & Cox, G. M. (1957). *Experimental designs* (2nd ed.). New York: John Wiley and Sons.

Cross, R. (1993). On the foundations of hysteresis in economic systems. *Economics and Philosophy, 9*, 53–74.

Ditto, P. H., Druley, J. A., Moore, K. A., Danks, J. H., & Smucker, W. D. (1996). Fates worse than death: The role of valued life activities in health-state evaluations. *Health Psychology, 15*, 332–343.

Edwards, A. L. (1957). The method of paired comparisons. In *Techniques of attitude scale construction*. (pp. 19–82). New York: Appleton-Century-Crofts.

Elston, R. C., & Grizzle, J. E. (1962). Estimation of time response curves and their confidence bands. *Biometrics, 18*, 148–159.

Francis, D. J., Fletcher, J. M., Stuebing, K. K., Davidson, K. C., & Thompson, N. M. (1992). Analysis of change: Modeling individual growth. In A. E. Kazdin (Ed.), *Methodological issues and strategies in clinical research*. (pp. 607–630). Washington, DC: American Psychological Association.

Freidlin, M., & Pfeiffer, R. (1998). A threshold estimation problem for processes with hysteresis. *Statistics and Probability Letters, 36*, 337–347.

Golembiewski, R. T., Billingsley, K., & Yeager, S. (1976). Measuring change and persistence in human affairs: Types of change generated by OLD designs. *Journal of Applied Behavioral Science, 12*, 133–157.

Granier, M. J., Green, S. B., & Armenakis, A. A. (1991). An experimental approach to evaluate methods to detect scale recalibration. *Educational and Psychological Measurements, 51*, 597–607.

Hoogstraten, J. (1982). The retrospective pretest in an educational training context. *Journal of Experimental Education, 50*, 200–204.

Hoogstraten, J. (1985). Influence of objective measures on self-reports in a retrospective pretest–posttest design. *Journal of Experimental Education, 53*, 207–210.

Howard, G. S., & Dailey, P. R. (1979). Response shift bias: A source of contamination of self-report measures. *Journal of Applied Psychology, 64*, 144–150.

Howard, G. S., Dailey, P. R., & Gulanick, N. A. (1979b). The feasibility of informed pretests in attenuating response-shift bias. *Applied Psychological Measurement, 3*, 481–494.

Howard, G. S., Millham, J., Slaten, S., & O'Donnell, L. (1981). Influence of subject response style effects on retrospective measures. *Applied Psychological Measurement, 5*, 89–100.

Howard, G. S., Ralph, K. M., Gulanick, N. A., Maxwell, S. E., Nance, S. W., & Gerber, S. K. (1979a). Internal invalidity in pretest–posttest self-report evaluations and a re-evaluation of retrospective pretests. *Applied Psychological Measurement, 3*, 1–23.

Howard, G. S., Schmeck, R. R., & Bray, J. H. (1979c). Internal invalidity in studies employing self-report instruments. A suggested remedy. *Journal of Educational Measurement, 16*, 129–135.

Jambon, B., & Johnson, K. I. (1997). Individual quality of life and clinical trials. *Quality of Life Newsletter, 1-2,* 16–17.

Jöreskog, K., & Sörbom, D. (1981). *LISREL V: Analysis of linear structural relationships by maximum likelihood and least square methods.* Uppsala, Sweden: University of Uppsala, Department of Statistics.

Kahneman, D., & Tversky, A. (1979). Prospect theory: An analysis of decision under risk. *Econometrica, 47,* 263–291.

Korth, B., & Tucker, L. (1975). The distribution of chance congruence coefficients from simulated data. *Psychometrika, 40,* 361–372.

Laird, N. M., & Ware, J. H. (1982). Random-effects models for longitudinal data. *Biometrics, 38,* 963–974.

Lechtenberg, R. (1988). *Multiple Sclerosis fact book.* Philadelphia: F. A. Davis Company.

Lenert, L. A., Morss, S., Goldstein, M. K., Bergen, M. R., Faustman, W. D., & Garber, A. M. (1997). Measurement of the validity of utility elicitations performed by computerized interview. *Medical Care, 35*(9), 915–920.

Levinson, W., Gordon, G., & Skeff, K. (1990). Retrospective versus actual pre-course self-assessments. *Evaluation Health Profession, 13,* 445–452.

Lindley, D. V., & Smith, A. F. M. (1972). Bayes estimates for the linear model. *Journal of the Royal Statistical Society Series, B 34,* 1–41.

Littel, R. C., Milliken, G. A., Stroup, W. W., & Wolfinger, R. D. (1996). *SAS System for mixed models.* Cary, NC: SAS Institute.

Mayergoyz, I. D. (1991). *Mathematical models of hysteresis.* New York: Springer-Verlag.

Nich, C., & Carroll, K. (1997). Now you see it, now you don't: A comparison of traditional versus random-effects regression models in the analysis of longitudinal follow-up data from a clinical trial. *Journal of Consulting and Clinical Psychology, 65,* 252–261.

Norman, P., & Parker, S. (1996). The interpretation of change in verbal reports: Implications for health psychology. *Psychology and Health, 11,* 301–314.

O'Boyle, C. A. (1994). The Schedule for the Evaluation of Individual Quality of Life (SEIQoL). *International Journal of Mental Health, 23,* 3–23.

O'Boyle, C. A., McGee, H., Hickey, A., O'Malley, K., & Joyce, C. R. B. (1992). Individual quality of life in patients undergoing hip replacement. *The Lancet, 339,* 1088–1091.

Powell, C. (1987). Quality of life measurement. *Journal of Medical Ethics, 12,* 222–223.

Randolph, W. A., & Elloy, D. F. (1989). How can OD consultants and researchers assess gamma change? A comparison of two analytic procedures. *Journal of Management, 15,* 633–648.

Rapkin, B. D., & Fischer, K. (1992). Personal goals of older adults: Issues in assessment and prediction. *Psychology and Aging, 7,* 127–137.

Rapkin, B. D., Smith, M. Y., Dumont, C. A., Palmer, S., & Cohen, S. (1994). Development of the idiographic functional status assessment: A measure of the personal goals and attainment activities of people with AIDS. *Psychology and Health, 9,* 111–129.

Rogosa, D., Brandt, D., & Zimowski, M. (1982). A growth curve approach to the measurement of change. *Psychological Bulletin, 92*(3), 726–748.

Ruta, D. A., Garratt, A. M., Leng, M., Russell, I. T., & MacDonald, L. M. (1994). A new approach to the measurement of quality of life: The patient-generated index. *Medical Care, 32,* 1109–1126.

Schmitt, N. (1982). The use of analysis of covariance structures to assess beta and gamma change. *Multivariate Behavioral Research, 17,* 343–358.

Schmitt, N., Pulakos, E., & Lieblein, A. (1984). Comparison of three techniques to assess group-level beta and gamma change. *Applied Psychological Measurement, 8,* 249–260.

Schwartz, C. E. (1996). Preference value assessment: Card sort approach. Copyrighted July 1996 by Frontier Science and Technology Foundation, Chestnut Hill, MA.

Schwartz, C. E. (1999). Teaching coping skills enhances quality of life more than peer support: Results of a randomized trial with multiple sclerosis patients. *Health Psychology, 18,* 211–220.

Schwartz, C. E., Cole, B. F., & Gelber, R. D. (1995a). Measuring patient-centered outcomes in neurologic disease: Extending the Q-TWiST methodology. *Archives of Neurology, 52,* 754–762.

Schwartz, C. E., Cole, B., Vickrey, B., & Gelber, R. (1995b). The Q-TWiST approach for assessing health-related quality of life in epilepsy. *Quality of Life Research, 4*, 135–141.

Schwartz, C. E., Coulthard-Morris, L., Cole, B., & Vollmer, T. (1997). The quality-of-life effects of Interferon-Beta-1b in multiple sclerosis: An Extended Q-TWiST analysis. *Archives of Neurology, 54*, 1475–1480.

Schwartz, C. E., & Lee, H. (1998). Response shift effects in a psychosocial randomized trial [Abstract]. *Psychosomatic Medicine, 60*, 115.

Schwartz, C. E., Peng, C. K., Lester, N., Daltroy, L., & Goldberger, A. (1998). Coping behavior in health and disease: Assessment with a card sort game. *Behavioral Medicine, 24*(1), 41–44.

Schwartz, C. E., & Sendor, M. (1999). Helping others helps oneself: Response shift effects in peer support. *Social Science and Medicine, 48*, 1563–1576.

Setterfield, M. (1997). Rapid growth and relative decline: Modelling macroeconomic dynamics with hysteresis. New York: St. Martin's Press.

Sheiner, L. B. (1985). Modeling pharmacodynamics: Parametric and nonparametric approaches. Variability. In M. Rowland et al. (Eds.), *Drug therapy: Description, estimation, and control*. New York: Raven Press.

Skeff, K. M., Stratos, G. A., & Bergen, M. R. (1992). Evaluation of a medical faculty development program. *Evaluation Health Profession, 15*, 350–366.

Soetikno, R. M., Mrad, R., Pao, V., & Lenert, L. A. (1997). Quality of life research on the internet: Feasibility and potential biases in patients with ulcerative colitis. *Journal of the American Medical Informatics Association 4*(6), 426–435.

Speer, D. C., & Greenbaum, P. E. (1995). Five methods for computing significant individual client change and improvement rates: Support for an individual growth curve approach. *Journal of Consulting and Clinical Psychology, 63*, 1044–1048.

Sprangers, M. A. G. (1988). Response shift and the retrospective pretest: On the usefulness of retrospective pretest–posttest designs in detecting training related response shifts. Het Instituut voor Onderzoek van het Onderwijs SVO, 's Gravenhage.

Sprangers, M. A. G. (1989). Response-shift bias in program evaluation. *Impact Assessment Bulletin, 7*, 153–166.

Sprangers, M. A. G. (1996). Response shift bias: A challenge to the assessment of patients' quality of life in cancer clinical trials. *Cancer Treatment Reviews, 22SA*, 55–62.

Sprangers, M. A. G., & van Dam, F. S. A. M. (1994, March). *Integrating response shift into health-related quality-of-life research: A first exploratory study.* Netherlands: The Netherlands Cancer Institute.

Sprangers, M. A. G., van Dam, F. S. A. M., Broersen, J., Lodder, L., Wever, L., Visser, M., Oosterveld, P., & Smets, E. M. (1999). Revealing response-shift in longitudinal research on fatigue: The use of Thentest approach. *Acta Oncologica, 38*, 709–718.

Sprangers, M. A. G., & Hoogstraten, J. (1987). Response-style effects, response-shift bias and a bogus-pipeline. *Psychological Reports, 61*, 579–585.

Sprangers, M. A. G., & Hoogstraten, J. (1989). Pretesting effects in retrospective pretest–posttest designs. *Journal of Applied Psychology, 74*, 265–272.

Sprangers, M. A. G., & Schwartz, C. E. (1999). Integrating response shift into health-related quality-of-life research: A theoretical model. *Social Science and Medicine, 48*, 1507–1515.

Stephenson, W. (1953). *The study of behavior*. Chicago: University of Chicago Press.

Stieglitz, R. D. (1990). Validatsstudien zum retrospetkiven Vortest in der Therapieforschung [Validity study into the retrospective pretest in therapy research]. *Zeitschrift fur Klinische Psychologie, 19*, 144–150.

Sugar, C. A., Strum, R., Lee, T. T., Sherborne, C. D., Olshen, R. A., Wells, K. B., & Lenert, L. A. (1998). Empirically defined health states for depression from the SF-12. *Health Services Research, 33*(4), 911–928.

Terborg, J. R., Maxwell, S. E., & Howard, G. S. (1980). Evaluating planned organizational change: A method for assessing alpha, beta and gamma change. *Academy of Management Review, 5*, 109–121.

Terborg, J. R., Maxwell, S. E., & Howard, G. S. (1982). On the measurement and control of beta change: Problems with the Bedeian, Armenakis, and Gibson technique. *Academy of Management Review, 7*, 292–295.

Thunedborg, K., Allerup, P., Bech, P., & Joyce, C. R. B. (1993). Development of the Repertory Grid for measurement of individual quality of life in clinical trials. *International Journal of Methods in Psychiatric Research, 3,* 45–56.

Torrance, G. W. (1986). Measurement of health state utilities for economic appraisal. *Journal of Health Economics, 5,* 1–30.

Willett, J. B., Ayoub, C. C., & Robinson, D. (1991). Using growth modeling to examine systematic differences in growth: An example of change in the functioning of families at risk of maladaptive parenting, child abuse, or neglect. *Journal of Consulting and Clinical Psychology, 59,* 38–47.

Willett, J. B., & Sayer, A. G. (1996). Cross-domain analyses of change over time: Combining growth modeling and covariance structure analysis. In G. A. Marcoulides & R. E. Schumacker (Eds.), *Advanced structural equation modeling: Issues and techniques.* Mahwah, NJ: Lawrence Erlbaum Associates.

Wittenborn, J. R. (1961). Contributions and current status of Q methodology. *Psychological Bulletin, 58,* 132–142.

Zmud, R., & Armenakis, A. A. (1978). Understanding of the measurement of change. *Academy of Management Review, 3,* 661–669.

7

Response Shift Effects on Patients' Evaluations of Health States: Sources of Artifact

Hilary A. Llewellyn-Thomas and Carolyn E. Schwartz

Approaches to Gathering Health State Evaluations

In health services research, the investigator often needs to obtain quantitative evaluations of different states of health from raters who are either experiencing or imagining these states. Such evaluations are used in health status indices, screening and monitoring care, clinical decision analysis, clinical trials, cost–utility analysis, or program evaluation (Berzon & Schumaker, 1994). First, descriptions of the relevant health states are prepared (Llewellyn-Thomas, 1996). A health state description is a paragraph consisting of different "attributes" (e.g., the ability to carry out self-care, the ability to carry out usual work activities, the intensity of a symptom like pain). Because each attribute can be represented at different levels, all the possible attribute and level combinations yield a set of different health state descriptions. In the full set, one description will approximate a particular individual's (or rater's) experienced health state, whereas the remaining descriptions represent imaginary health states.

Then, for each health state, the investigator elicits an evaluative score representing the rater's judgment of its overall desirability, or relative position on the good health–death continuum. The most common elicitation techniques are the standard gamble (von Neumann & Morgenstern, 1953), the time trade-off (Torrance, 1976), and the linear analogue scale (Hoepfl & Huber, 1978; Llewellyn-Thomas, Sutherland, Ciampi et al., 1984). The theoretical rationale underlying these techniques, their procedural details, and the issues regarding their use are treated in depth elsewhere (Froberg & Kane, 1989; Torrance, 1976). The focus of this chapter is on investigators who are interested primarily in the response shift

The work of National Health Scholar Hilary A. Llewellyn-Thomas was supported by the National Health Research & Development Program, Canada. The work of Carolyn E. Schwartz was supported in part by Agency for Health Care Policy and Research Grant RO1 HSO8582–03.

phenomenon. These investigators wish to identify when raters actually change their internal standards of measurement, change their values, or redefine their conceptualization of the experienced or imagined health states (see chapters 1 and 6). To do this, they elicit evaluations from the same raters on more than one occasion using different kinds of longitudinal research designs.

One design involves following patients to see whether evaluations of their experienced health state change according to actual disease- or treatment-related alterations in their objective health status. Objective health status might actually worsen across time, whereas patients' evaluations might remain constant or even improve. Another design involves obtaining evaluations of a set of imagined health states on more than one occasion, to see whether they are stable in spite of actual disease- or treatment-related alterations in the raters' own health status. Objective health status might actually worsen across time, but the evaluations of the imagined states might also change. A third design involves asking for an anticipatory evaluation of an imagined health state that patients may encounter later, then obtaining this evaluation again when the state becomes a reality. The subjective evaluations might change when the state is no longer imaginary.

In all of these situations, the investigator might conclude that response shift has occurred, then try to tease out the relative contribution of each of the three components. However, the elicitation procedures themselves can either prevent the investigator from clearly identifying which component is operating or can induce covert effects that could be mistaken for actual changes in the internal standards of measurement, for actual change in values, or for an actual redefinition of health. This chapter provides an organizational framework for these obscuring and artifactual effects, given different kinds of health state descriptions and different ways of obtaining evaluations. For investigators studying the three components of true response shift, this framework could help them anticipate these effects and guide appropriate study design modifications. Each of the three components is considered separately. In each section, actual components are defined, the obscuring or artifactual effects that interfere with clear detection are outlined, and ways to avoid such effects are indicated. Change in the internal standards of measurement is treated in somewhat more detail, because more is currently known about the effects to which change is susceptible.

Changes in Internal Standards of Measurement

Actual Changes in Internal Standards

Actual change in raters' internal standards of measurement occurs when, either consciously or unconsciously, they alter their internal point of reference while assigning evaluative scores to health states, which, in turn, induces recalibration of their internal measurement scale. The direction and degree of actual change depend on whether raters are asked to evaluate their own experienced health state or a set of imagined health states and on whether the study design stimulates self-referenced comparisons or social comparisons (Llewellyn-Thomas et al., 1991; Redelmeier, Guyatt, & Goldstein, 1996).

Self-referenced comparisons. Actual changes in internal standards can be induced by either prospective or retrospective self-referenced comparisons. Prospectively, an individual experiences a health state that was previously purely imaginary. Cross-sectional studies imply that an experienced health state is evaluated more highly than is an imaginary one (Sackett & Torrance, 1978). One longitudinal study provided more detailed designs of qualitative changes in health status evaluation as a function of reference point. Patients provided evaluations for imaginary health states, and evaluations were re-elicited when the patients actually entered one of the states (Llewellyn-Thomas, Sutherland, & Thiel, 1993). Increments appeared when the patients entered states at the more severe end of the health–illness continuum, but evaluations for health states of mild to moderate severity remained comparable.

Conversely, other research has documented that when an individual provided an evaluation for an experienced health state, then moved out of that state and reevaluated it retrospectively, his or her evaluative score changed (Redelmeier & Kahneman, 1996). Kahneman and Tversky (1983) argued that the dynamics of rapid adaptation (Brickman & Campbell, 1971) account for this process. It is unknown whether shifts in self-referenced evaluations interact with other key aspects of the raters' experiences. These aspects include whether a rater expected to end up in the health state, as well as the direction and degree of the difference between expectation and actuality (Llewellyn-Thomas, Thiel, & McGreal, 1992).

Social comparisons. Actual changes in the internal standards of measurement also may be induced by social comparisons. Suppose the primary objective is to assess the stability of evaluations for experienced health states when there has been no objective change in the rater's overall health status. However, suppose that, in the interest of serving a secondary research objective, the investigator also asked for evaluations of some imagined health states just prior to the second self-evaluations. Respondents may focus on those who seem better off and actually change their internal standard of measurement in a way that exaggerates this perceived difference. Their subsequent evaluative score for their own state may thus be lowered. The actual change could occur in the opposite direction if the raters focus on those who seem to be worse off.

Avoiding Artifactual Effects

When it is important to detect actual changes in internal standards of measurement, the investigator must be able to differentiate it from artifactually induced effects that mimic such change. The three commonly used scaling techniques can themselves generate such effects, depending on their frames, sequences, and scalar end points.

Framing effects. Framing occurs with different presentations of probabilistically identical information (e.g., 80% survival rate versus 20% death rate). Different frames induce changes in the reference point used to judge an outcome as a gain or loss (Kahneman & Tversky, 1982, 1983; Tversky & Kahneman, 1981). This in turn can induce apparent preference reversals (Kahneman & Tversky, 1982; McNeil, Pauker, Sox, & Tversky, 1982; O'Connor, 1989; O'Connor et al., 1985), which could be misinterpreted as actual change in internal standards of measurement. To avoid stimulating this cognitive illusion, the investigator interested in actual change in internal standards would use a neutral frame during value elicitation. In a neutral frame, both the positive (gains) and negative (losses) aspects of the elicitation task are described. Thus, the probabilities of both perfect health and death (the traditional lottery outcomes used in the standard gamble), or both the survival time and the time lost (the traditional trade-off used in the time trade-off) would be presented (Llewellyn-Thomas, McGreal, & Thiel, 1995).

Sequence effects. The sequences followed when obtaining evaluations can create anchoring effects. Anchoring effects occur when the evaluation elicited by the first stimulus systematically skews the evaluations assigned to subsequent stimuli (Tversky & Kahneman, 1974). Thus, variations in sequence can inadvertently induce changes in raters' judgments of the relative positions of different health states on the underlying preference scale, which could be misinterpreted as evidence of actual change in internal standards of measurement.

Different kinds of sequences can generate an anchoring effect. First, overall (i.e., holistic) evaluations can be affected when sequences differ—for example, from the least to the most preferred, or vice versa (Llewellyn-Thomas et al., 1982). Second, when seeking the indifference point in the time trade-off or the standard gamble, different results could be obtained if the interviewer took the rater from one end of the time or probability scale toward the other, for example, from less to more survival time, from high to low risk of death, or vice versa (Lenert, Flowers, Goldstein, & Garber, 1995; Percy & Llewellyn-Thomas, 1995). Third, anchoring occurs when different techniques appear in particular sequences. For example, the elicitation of standard gamble utilities may subsequently affect linear analogue scores (Llewellyn-Thomas, Sutherland, Tibshirani, et al., 1984). These potential anchoring effects can be offset by randomizing the sequences of health states, scaling steps, and evaluative techniques wherever possible.

Scalar end point effects. When a response scale's end points are defined, effects that could be misinterpreted as evidence of change in internal standards of measurement can also be induced. It has been argued (Stevens, 1966, 1971) that raters do not accurately represent their discriminative judgments on interval response scales because they spread out ratings for stimuli that are actually similar and rate similarly those that are quite different, in order to use each scale interval equally often. Kaplan and Ernst's (1983) test of this argument suggests that this bias is more likely when the end points of the rating scale are poorly defined. Further work implied that, when the scale end points are systematically varied, raters tend not to make appropriate revisions to the numerical values they assign to imagined health states (Llewellyn-Thomas et al., 1982; Sutherland, Dunn, & Boyd, 1983). Taken together, these results suggest that the investigator interested in actual change in internal standards of measurement should ensure that the response continuum is made clear to participants and that health states specific to the clinical problem are used as the scalar end points.

A side note is necessary here, because purists may challenge the recommendation to use health states specific to the clinical problem as scalar end points. The traditional use of perfect health and death as scalar end points came about in order to make across-disease comparisons of evaluative scores. However, when disease-specific evaluative scores—rather than across-disease comparisons—are of primary interest, it would be acceptable to use the best (i.e., highest functioning, symptom-free) and the worst (i.e., lowest functioning, severe-symptom) states as scalar end points instead (Llewellyn-Thomas, 1996; Llewellyn-Thomas, Sutherland, Ciampi, et al., 1984; Llewellyn-Thomas, Williams, Levy, & Naylor, 1996). This strategy gives three advantages to the investigator interested in actual change in internal standards.

First, if death is used as an end point when non-life-threatening health states are evaluated, the resultant strong aversive attitude will generate skewed distributions that hide actual change in internal standards. Second, when the rater is evaluating his or her experienced disease-specific health state (e.g., angina) but also has comorbidity (e.g., arthritis), the exercise is likely to generate confounded evaluative scores (reflecting attitudes toward not only angina but also the comorbid arthritic state) if perfect health is used as an end point (Nichol, Llewellyn-Thomas, Naylor, & Thiel, 1996). Third, because attitudes toward death and comorbidity can shift with time, these end point effects may be further confounded, which would make it even more difficult to identify actual change in internal standards of measurement.

Given these arguments, investigators may choose to use health states that are specific to the clinical problem as scalar end points. Subsequent across-disease comparisons can be achieved by using a triangulation design that permits later transformation of the elicited scores. In this design, after the health states of interest are evaluated relative to the best and worst states, the best and worst states are themselves evaluated relative to the traditional perfect health and death outcome states. Then, using the axiom of substitutability, the original score for the health states of interest are revised to reflect their inferred evaluation relative to perfect health and death (Nichol et al., 1996). Thus, triangulated designs can control for end point effects that could distort actual change in internal standards and also can permit subsequent across-disease applications.

Changes in Values

Actual Changes in Values

As has been noted, a health state description incorporates different attributes. Actual changes in values occur when, either consciously or unconsciously, raters modify the relative importance of each attribute's contribution toward their judgment of the state's overall desirability. The detection of these actual changes in values is subject to obscuring and artifactual effects.

Avoiding Obscuring Effects

Suppose the objective is to assess the across-time stability of evaluations for experienced or imagined health states. Suppose also that the investigator elects to use a "holistic" strategy, which involves obtaining single overall evaluative scores for the health states of interest. Suppose further that the holistic scores appear either highly stable or systematically variable. On the one hand, the stability may be spurious. The rater may actually shift the relative weights ascribed to each individual attribute, but these shifts are mutually cancelled when the rater provides overall scores. On the other hand, the systematic change may be real and predominantly driven by shifts in the weight ascribed to one or more attributes. In either case, given the overall scores alone, the locus, direction, and degree of these attribute shifts cannot be pinpointed; the investigator interested in actual changes in attribute importance has been handicapped by the initial data collection strategy. This problem could be anticipated when the protocols for collecting evaluations of imagined or experienced health states are first being designed.

The investigator assessing the stability of evaluations for imagined states could deliberately use an appropriate factorial or semi-orthogonal design to guide the construction of the health states (Addelman, 1962). With this strategy, the levels of the constituent attributes are systematically varied at the time of data collection so that, later, regression modeling techniques can be applied to the entire set of observed holistic scores (Etezadi-Amoli & Ciampi, 1983). These models can indirectly reveal the respondent's policy of weighing and combining the attributes when making his or her holistic judgments (Slovic & Lichtenstein, 1971), given subsequent careful assessments of the fit of the derived model (Boyle & Torrance, 1984). This modeling could be done at test and retest to determine whether there has been a shift in the constellation of weights ascribed to the individual attributes.

Investigators assessing the stability of scores for an experienced health state can anticipate the interpretive problem by using an elicitation technique that makes explicit the attitude toward each attribute. For each rater, individual attribute weights are separately and directly quantified with a "decomposed" strategy in which evaluative scores are collected one attribute at a time (Hoepfl & Huber, 1978; Edwards, 1971, 1977; Keeney, 1977; Keeney & Raiffa, 1976). These weights are subsequently aggregated to yield an overall score for the entire health state description, although the assumed form of the aggregation model, that is, whether it is additive or multiplicative, must be carefully considered (Etezadi-Amoli & Ciampi, 1983). These directly obtained attribute weights would be collected at both test and retest times, to reveal explicitly whether there has been a shift in the constellation of weights ascribed to the individual attributes. This is often the most efficient way of proceeding for imagined health states as well, especially when the number of attributes and levels yields so many combinations that holistic assessment would be prohibitively time-consuming (Boyle & Torrance, 1984).

Avoiding Artifactual Effects

Thus, the evaluative strategy determines whether it will be possible to explore for changes in the relative importance of the attributes. Suppose the investigator has carried out this anticipatory planning. He or she should also realize that the attribute presentation can itself generate effects that mimic an actual shift in an attribute's importance. These artifacts could arise from the format used to outline the attributes, the manner in which the attributes are framed, and the sequence of the attributes.

Format effects. Written descriptions can be constructed in either point or narrative format. In point format, the attributes are merely labeled in lists, which may make it easier to consider several attributes at once. It may be easier, however, to identify personally with a narrative format, in which the health state is described in a short paragraph. It is largely unknown whether using different formats in the same study makes some attributes more salient than others and consequently induces spurious changes in their relative importance (Nisbett & Ross, 1980). Furthermore, this artifactual effect may be differentially manifested depending on whether linear analogue, time trade-off, or standard gamble is used (Llewellyn-Thomas, Sutherland, Ciampi, et al., 1984). Thus, the investigator who wants clearly interpretable evidence of actual change in attribute importance would keep both format and technique constant.

Framing effects. As has been noted earlier, different probabilistic frames can change the judgment of an outcome as a possible gain or loss. In a similar vein, the attributes in a health state description could be inadvertently framed. For example, the same level of functional ability could be presented positively ("You are still able to . . .") or negatively ("You are no longer able to . . ."). Variations in attribute framing could make some more salient than others and consequently induce spurious changes in attribute importance. To avoid this artifact, the investigator would avoid switching from one frame to another or would use a balanced frame to describe the various functional levels in each attribute. A balanced frame is a way of presenting information in a format that includes both positive and negative perspectives. This format can be used for both quantitative information (e.g., "The chance of five year survival is 85%; the chance of death within five years is 15%.") and qualitative information (e.g., "Unable to [functional disability]; able to [functional capability]").

Sequence effects. Even with the consistent use of format and frame, attribute sequence can induce effects that could be misinterpreted as actual change in attribute importance. When decomposed evaluations are being elicited, one may create systematic anchoring effects if positive attributes always appear before the negative, or vice versa. When holistic evaluations are to be obtained, factorial or semi-orthogonal designs are used to develop a set of health states reflecting a full range of attribute levels. However, if the design is inattentively used—for example, in a manner that always arranges the attribute levels from least to most dysfunctional—the subsequent holistic evaluations could also be subject to anchoring effects (Llewellyn-Thomas et al., 1982). These possible effects can be minimized by counterbalancing the sequences in which positive and negative attributes are presented, in either decomposed or holistic strategies.

Changes in Conceptualization

Actual Changes in Conceptualization

Actual changes in conceptualization occur when a rater redefines the personal meaning of the different attributes of (his or her) health. This redefinition can occur either consciously or unconsciously. In the interest of constructing a particular kind of health state description for a particular research purpose, the investigator has to make particular decisions about study design (Feeny, Furlong, Boyle, & Torrance, 1995). These early design steps may inadvertently lead to a data collection strategy that will preclude the clear observation of actual attribute redefinition.

Avoiding Obscuring Effects

The earliest design step involves deciding on the range of attributes to be incorporated into the health state descriptions. The investigator needs to consider whether, given the study purpose, the health state descriptions should incorporate a narrow (e.g., disease-specific) or wide (e.g., generic) range of attributes. The next step involves choosing a particular procedure for attribute selection. The relevant attributes could be identified from published empirical work, from the impressions of expert clinicians, from focus groups, or from surveys of patients. Then, after a list of possible attributes has been created, what algorithm will be used to select the key attributes? One could elect to either (a) apply an explicit conceptual framework regarding the definition of health, (b) retain only clinically modifiable attributes and set others aside, or (c) retain only those attributes for which cost implications can be determined.

Finally, there remains the issue of whose point of view counts when identifying the initial list of attributes and deciding on which to include and to delete. Clinicians, policy makers, consumers, and patients may have different points of view. The answers to all of these questions depend on the research purpose guiding the particular investigation, as well as on the investigator's rationale for using the point of view of one group to draw inferences that will have implications for a different group. Hence, these decisions are unavoidable. However, at the same time, they may inadvertently make it very difficult to detect actual attribute redefinition.

An example may help illustrate this argument. Suppose we are interested in evaluating the effects of treatment, and we plan to proceed by comparing pre- and posttreatment self-assessments of patients receiving, for example, total joint replacement surgery. Suppose we had elected to use disease-specific attributes, had decided to focus on attributes that are most likely to be affected by the surgical intervention, and had derived these from the existing clinical literature in arthritis. Thus, we might proceed by (a) asking candidates for surgery to report whether they currently experience no, mild, moderate, or severe distress in, for example, six disease-specific dimensions (pain, stiffness, difficulty doing home or work activities, difficulty doing self-care activities, restrictions in leisure activities, and emotional distress due to arthritis); (b) using these six self-ratings to create an individualized descriptive paragraph summarizing each patient's current presurgical arthritis-specific health state; and then (c) asking the patient to provide an overall evaluation of the relative desirability of this state (Llewellyn-Thomas, Arshinoff, Bell, Williams, & Naylor, 1998). These steps would be repeated at a selected time point after surgery (e.g., one year), and the overall evaluations obtained after surgery would be compared to those provided prior to surgery.

Note how attribute redefinition could become an issue in this example. The assumption that it is appropriate to use these six disease-specific attributes may be valid at the presurgical time point. However, by the time the patient reaches the one-year postsurgical time point, new attributes —for example, the patient's satisfaction with his or her relationship with the physician—may loom larger in the patient's mind and spill into the overall evaluation of the postsurgical health state. Thus, although the second overall evaluation could move in the anticipated direction (i.e., the score could be higher, reflecting the benefits of surgery), it would be a composite of the actual improvement incurred in the six attributes of interest and the spillover of unidentified attributes newly introduced into the judgment task (Nisbett & Ross, 1980).

One way of exploring whether the health state has been consciously redefined by the patient in this hidden way is explicitly to seek qualitative reports from the patient (in this example, particularly at the postsurgical interview) about whether the attributes are still relevant as well as about whether new attributes should be incorporated in the health state descriptions. This additional data collection phase would need to be formally built into the original study protocol, and time and funds would need to be allocated for the qualitative data analysis. The interpretation of the qualitative data is also tempered by the limitations of this approach, because it cannot capture unconscious redefinition of the constituent elements of the health state of interest (see chapter 6).

Conclusion

In this chapter we have presented a methodologic framework for designing evaluative studies that will not obscure or artifactually affect actual changes in internal standards of measurement, in values, and in the conceptualization of health. This framework is summarized in Table 7.1. First, the clear identification of actual changes in internal standards of measurement can be artifactually affected by different probabilistic time frames, different elicitation sequences, and the use of the traditional scalar end points. To avoid this, the investigator should consider using neutral frames, random sequences, and disease-specific scalar end points.

Second, the identification of actual changes in values can be handicapped by obscuring and artifactual effects. Obscuring will occur with the exclusive use of a holistic evaluative strategy. If a holistic strategy is necessary, the investigator could use appropriate factorial or semi-orthogonal designs when constructing the original set of health states, then use regression modeling to analyze the evaluative scores. If a holistic strategy can be set aside, a decomposed evaluative strategy entirely avoids the obscuring effect. Artifactual effects can be induced by using different formats to present attributes, different attribute frames, and different attribute sequences, all of which can alter the perceived salience of attributes. These artifactual effects can interfere with the clear identification of actual change in the attributes' relative importance; the investigator wishing to identify such change would use a consistent attribute format, balanced attribute frames, and randomized attribute sequences.

Third, the clear identification of reconceptualizations of health can be obscured when early design decisions about attribute range and the process of attribute selection rest on covert assumptions that do not maintain their validity across time. To offset this obscuring effect, careful thought should go into the collection of qualitative data to determine whether the attributes are still relevant to the raters and whether new attributes should be incorporated into the health state descriptions.

Investigating the response shift phenomenon could help us address fundamental and applied research problems in health care decision making. Fundamental work could lead to deeper insights into how evaluations are formed and modified by time and the illness experience. Those insights

Table 7.1. A Framework for Differentiating Between Actual Response Shift and Obscuring or Artifactual Effects

Response shift component	Operationalization	Sources of obscuring or artifactual effects	Study design modifications
Changes in internal standards of measurement	Recalibration of respondents' internal measurement scale	*Artifactual effects* Framing of scaling techniques Sequences in scaling techniques End points in scaling techniques	Use neutral probabilistic/time frames. Randomize sequences of health states, scaling steps, evaluative techniques. Use disease-specific "best" and "worst" scalar end points, then triangulate.
Changes in values	Change in relative importance ascribed to constituent attributes	*Obscuring effects* "Holistic" assessment strategy *Artifactual effects* Format of attributes Frame of attributes Sequences of attributes	Use factorial or semi-orthogonal design to construct health states, with subsequent regression modeling. Use "decomposed" assessment strategy. Keep point form or narrative format consistent. Use balanced functional/dysfunctional attribute frames. Counterbalance sequences of attributes.
Changes in conceptualization	Redefinition of constituent attributes of health state of interest	*Obscuring effects* Early design decisions about range of attributes and about process of attribute selection	Collect qualitative data to determine 1. whether attributes are still relevant. 2. whether new attributes should be incorporated into health state descriptions.

could then guide investigations into important clinical issues. One issue is how best to provide patients with information about probable changes in their evaluation of future health states, without covertly influencing the direction of their decisions. Another issue is how to communicate, in ethically appropriate ways, information about actual changes in patients' self-evaluations to health care professionals and family members, because this information could be relevant to their involvement in patients' health care decisions. To study these issues well, it will be crucial to differentiate between actual response shift and obscuring or artifactual effects induced by the process of value elicitation. Thus, the framework described herein may facilitate the clear emergence of response shift as an informative and promising phenomenon.

References

Addelman, S. (1962). Orthogonal main effect plans for symmetrical factorial experiments. *Technometrics, 4,* 21–46.

Berzon, R., & Schumaker, S. (1994). Evaluating health-related quality of life measures for cross-national research. *Drug Information Journal, 28,* 63–70.

Boyle, M. H., & Torrance, G. W. (1984). Developing multiattribute health indexes. *Medical Care, 22,* 1045–1057.

Brickman, P., & Campbell, D. T. (1971). Hedonic relativism and planning the good society. In M. H. Appley (Ed.), *Adaptation-level theory: A symposium* (p. 287). New York: Academic Press.

Edwards, W. (1971). Social utilities. *The Engineering Economist: Summer Symposium Series, 6,* 119–129.

Edwards W. (1977). How to use multiattribute utility measurement for social decision making. *IEEE Transactions on Systems, Man, and Cybernetics, SMC-7,* 326–340.

Etezadi-Amoli, J., & Ciampi, A. (1983). Simultaneous parameter estimation for the multiplicative multiattribute utility model. *Organizational Behaviour and Human Performance, 32,* 232–248.

Feeny, D., Furlong, W., Boyle M., & Torrance, G. W. (1995). Multiattribute health status classification systems: Health Utilities Index. *PharmacoEconomics, 7,* 490–502.

Froberg, D. G., & Kane, R. L. (1989). Methodology for measuring health-state preferences: II. Scaling methods. *Journal of Clinical Epidemiology, 42,* 459–471.

Hoepfl, R. T., & Huber, G. P. (1978). A study of self-explicated utility models. *Behavioural Science, 15,* 408–413.

Kahneman, D., & Tversky, A. (1982). The psychology of preferences. *Scientific American, 246,* 160–173.

Kahneman, D., & Tversky, A. (1983). Choices, values, and frames. *American Psychologist, 39,* 341–350.

Kaplan, R. M., & Ernst, J. A. (1983). Do category rating scales produce biased preference weights for a health index? *Medical Care, 21,* 193–207.

Keeney, R. L. (1977). The art of assessing multiattribute utility functions. *Organizational Behaviour and Human Performance, 19,* 267–310.

Keeney, R. L, & Raiffa, H. (1976). *Decisions with multiple objectives: Preference and value trade-offs.* New York: Wiley.

Lenert, L. A., Flowers, C., Goldstein, M. K., & Garber, A. M. (1995). Effect of method of search for subjects' indifference point on the reliability and validity of standard gamble utilities. *Medical Decision Making, 15*(Abstract), 430.

Llewellyn-Thomas, H. A. (1996). Health state descriptions: Purposes, issues, a proposal. *Medical Care, 34,* DS109-DS118.

Llewellyn-Thomas, H. A., Arshinoff, R., Bell, M., Williams, J. I., & Naylor, C. D. (1998). In the queue for total joint replacement: Patients' perspectives on waiting times. *Journal of Evaluation in Clinical Practice, 4,* 63–74.

Llewellyn-Thomas, H. A., McGreal, M. J., & Thiel, E. C. (1995). Cancer patients' decision making and trial entry preferences: The effects of "framing" information about short-term toxicity and long-term survival. *Medical Decision Making, 15,* 4–12.

Llewellyn-Thomas, H. A., Sutherland, H. J., Ciampi, A., Etezadi-Amoli, J., Boyd, N. F., & Till, J. E. (1984). The assessment of values in laryngeal cancer: Reliability of measurement methods. *Journal of Chronic Diseases, 37,* 283–291.

Llewellyn-Thomas, H. A., Sutherland, H. J., & Thiel, E. C. (1993). Do patients' evaluations of a future health state change when they actually enter that state? *Medical Care, 31,* 1002–1012.

Llewellyn-Thomas, H. A., Sutherland, H. J., Tibshirani, R., Ciampi, A., Till, J. E., & Boyd, N. F. (1982). The measurement of patients' values in medicine. *Medical Care, 20,* 449–462.

Llewellyn-Thomas, H. A., Sutherland, H. J., Tibshirani, R., Ciampi, A., Till, J. E., & Boyd, N. F. (1984). Describing health states: Methodologic issues in obtaining values for health states. *Medical Care, 22,* 543–552.

Llewellyn-Thomas, H. A., Sutherland, H. J., Tritchler, D. L., Lockwood, G., Till, J. E., Ciampi, A., Scott, J. F., Lickley, L. A., & Fish, E. B. (1991). Benign and malignant breast disease: The relationship between women's health status and health values. *Medical Decision Making, 11,* 180–188.

Llewellyn-Thomas, H. A., Thiel, E. C., & McGreal, M. J. (1992). Cancer patients' evaluations of their current health states: The influences of expectations, comparisons, actual health status, and mood. *Medical Decision Making, 12,* 115–122.

Llewellyn-Thomas, H. A., Williams, J. I., Levy, L., & Naylor, C. D. (1996). Benign prostatic hyperplasia (BPH): Using a trade-off technique to assess patients' treatment preferences. *Medical Decision Making, 16,* 162–172.

McNeil, B. J., Pauker, S. G., Sox, H. C., & Tversky, A. (1982). On the elicitation of preferences for alternative therapies. *New England Journal of Medicine, 306,* 1259–1262.

von Neumann, J., & Morgenstern, O. (1953). *The theory of games and economic behavior* (3rd ed.). New York: Wiley.

Nichol, G., Llewellyn-Thomas, H. A., Naylor, C. D., & Thiel, E. C. (1996). The relationship between cardiac functional capacity and patients' symptom-specific utilities for angina: Some findings and methodologic lessons. *Medical Decision Making, 16,* 78–85.

Nisbett, R., & Ross, L. (1980). *Human inference: Strategies and shortcomings of social judgment* (pp. 43–62). Englewood Cliffs, NJ: Prentice-Hall.

O'Connor, A. (1989). Effects of framing and level of probability on patients' preferences for cancer chemotherapy. *Journal of Clinical Epidemiology, 42,* 119–126.

O'Connor, A. M. C., Boyd, N. F., Tritchler, D. L., Kriukov, Y., Sutherland, H., & Till, J. E. (1985). Eliciting preferences for alternative cancer drug treatments: The influence of framing, medium, and rater variables. *Medical Decision Making, 4,* 453–463.

Percy, M. E., & Llewellyn-Thomas, H. A. (1995). Assessing preferences about the DNR order: Does it depend on how you ask? *Medical Decision Making, 15,* 209–216.

Redelmeier, D. A., Guyatt, G. H., & Goldstein, R. S. (1996). Assessing the minimal important difference in symptoms: A comparison of two techniques. *Journal of Clinical Epidemiology, 49,* 1215–1219.

Redelmeier, D. A., & Kahneman, D. (1996). Patients' memories of painful medical treatments: Real-time and retrospective evaluations of two minimally invasive procedures. *Pain, 66,* 3–8.

Sackett, D. L., & Torrance, G. W. (1978). The utility of different health states as perceived by the general public. *Journal of Chronic Diseases, 31,* 697–704.

Slovic, P., & Lichtenstein, S. (1971). Comparison of Bayesian and regression approaches to the study of information processing in judgement. *Organizational Behaviour and Human Performance, 6,* 649–744.

Stevens, S. S. (1966). A metric for the social consensus. *Science, 151,* 530–541.

Stevens, S. S. (1971). Issues in psychophysical measurement. *Psychological Review, 78,* 426–450.

Sutherland, H. J., Dunn, V., & Boyd, N. F. (1983). Measurement of values for states of health with linear analogue scales. *Medical Decision Making, 3,* 477–487.

Torrance, G. W. (1976). Social preference for health states: An empirical evaluation of three measurement techniques. *Socio-Economic Planning Sciences, 10,* 129–136.

Tversky, A., & Kahneman, D. (1974). Judgment under uncertainty: Heuristics and biases. *Science, 185,* 1124–1131.

Tversky, A., & Kahneman, D. (1981). The framing of decisions and the psychology of choice. *Science, 211,* 453–458.

8

Measuring Response Shift Using the Schedule for Evaluation of Individual Quality of Life

Ciaran A. O'Boyle, Hannah M. McGee, and John P. Browne

The subjective, dynamic nature of quality of life (QOL) creates significant difficulties for its measurement (Hunt, 1997; Joyce, O'Boyle, & McGee, 1999), and research in this area has produced a number of apparently contradictory findings. First, there is the discrepancy between observer or proxy ratings of QOL and those of the individual concerned (Sprangers & Aaronson, 1992). Second, the expected deterioration in QOL often does not occur, even in cases of serious illness, injury, or aging (Browne et al., 1994; Evans, 1991; Kreitler, Samario, Rapoport, Kreitler, & Algor, 1993). Third, serious illness can actually result in an increase in patient satisfaction and QOL (Andrykowski, Brady, & Hunt, 1993).

These contradictory findings highlight the dynamic nature of QOL and the importance of studying response shift when assessing changes in subjective ratings. Golembiewsky, Billingsley, and Yeager (1976) had suggested three types of changes that may occur in the subjective assessments. Alpha change involves a variation in the objective level of some existential state, given a constantly calibrated measuring instrument related to a constant conceptual domain. Beta change involves a variation in the level of some existential state, complicated by the fact that some intervals of the measurement continuum associated with a constant conceptual state have been recalibrated. Gamma change involves a redefinition or reconceptualization of some domain, which results in a major change in the perspective or frame of reference.

A number of authors have recently attempted to define response shift in a health care context and to suggest methods that might be appropriate for its measurement. The Golembiewsky approach has recently provided the basis for a detailed discussion of the dynamic nature of QOL (Allison, Locker, & Feine, 1997) and has been further developed by Schwartz and Sprangers (see chapters 1 and 6). These latter authors have defined response shift as a change in the meaning of one's self-evaluation of a target construct as the result of (a) a change in one's internal standards of measurement (scale recalibration), (b) a change in one's values (i.e., importance of component domains constituting the target construct), or (c) a redefinition of the target construct (reconceptualization).

The phenomenological approach to QOL focuses on the unique experiences of the individual whereby QOL can be defined as that which the individual determines it to be (for a review, see Joyce et al., 1999). The individual's perspective is likely to change with, for example, the passage of time or as a result of a major illness or life event. The problem for an external observer is that the individual's perception of an event rather than the event itself is likely to be the crucial factor in altering their judgment of QOL. The phenomenological perspective has resulted in the development of a number of measures of QOL that seek to incorporate the unique views of the individual. These include the Patient Generated Index (Ruta, Garratt, Leng, Russell, & McDonald, 1994), the Repertory Grid Technique (Dunbar, Stoker, Hodges, & Beaumont, 1992; Thunedborg, Allerup, Bech, & Joyce, 1993), the QOL Index (Ferrans & Powers, 1995), and utility measures of QOL that, although having a different emphasis, incorporate the individual perspective (Bennett & Torrance, 1996). One measure adopting this approach is the Schedule for the Evaluation of Individual Quality of Life or SEIQOL (O'Boyle et al., 1993). The purpose of this chapter is to describe how the SEIQOL may be applied to measuring some elements of response shift.

SEIQOL

The SEIQOL is based on judgment analysis, a well-established technique for modeling judgments (Cooksey, 1996). It measures three elements of QOL: (a) cues—the areas of life that are most important to the respondent's QOL, (b) levels—how the respondent is currently doing in each of these areas, and (c) weights—the relative importance of each of these cues to the respondent's overall QOL. The SEIQOL consists of a number of stages: cue elicitation, assessment of cue levels, derivation of cue weights by means of judgment analysis, and calculation of a global QOL score known as the SEIQOL index score.

During a structured interview, respondents are first asked to think about their lives and nominate the five areas of life (cues) that they consider most important to their overall QOL. The number of cues was set at five because research indicates that most people experience difficulty in making judgments requiring combining information from a larger number of cues (Stewart, 1988). The meaning of each cue is recorded together with the label the respondent uses for each cue. For example, different respondents may use "religion" as a cue label, but it can have various meanings: a spiritual activity, a social activity (meeting friends at services), or a physical activity reflecting mobility (being able to walk to services). The definition is important for subsequent understanding of what the respondent intended by the cue label and for aggregating cues from a number of respondents.

Respondents then rate their current status on each cue against a vertical visual analogue scale, labeled at the upper and lower extremities by the terms "as good as could possibly be" and "as bad as could possibly be," respectively. The interviewer generates a profile using a bar chart with five columns representing the five ratings, and the respondent is asked to consider this overall profile and rate a global QOL on a horizontal visual analogue scale. The cue levels are used subsequently to generate a profile of the respondent's QOL.

To quantify the relative importance of each cue, judgment analysis is used. Judgment analysis, which is also known as *policy capturing*, has been widely used in studies of judgment and decision making. It externalizes the manner in which a person makes a judgment or decision (their judgment policy), by using statistical methods to derive an algebraic model of the judgment process. The goal is to quantify the relationships between a person's judgment and the information, or cues, used to make that judgment (Cooksey, 1996). The theoretical foundations for judgment analysis lie in Brunswick's lens model (Brunswick, 1956) and in social judgment theory (Brehmer & Joyce, 1988; Hammond, Stewart, Brehmer, & Steinmann, 1975).

The respondent is presented with 30 randomly generated profiles of hypothetical subjects labeled using their five previously chosen cues and is asked to rate the global QOL for each profile. It is estimated that 10 cases are required to derive a judgment policy with three uncorrelated cues and another 5 cases for each additional cue; thus 20 cases are required for five cues (Stewart, 1988). Ten additional repeated cases are included in order to estimate internal reliability. The relative weight attached by the respondent to each of the cues in judging global QOL is calculated by multiple regression (Executive Decision Services, 1986). One of the advantages of the method is that it can measure the relative cue weights that may be unknown to the participant (precognitive).

Because time and resources may be limited in certain clinical situations, a simpler direct method of measuring cue weights, the SEIQOL–DW, has been developed (Browne, O'Boyle, McGee, McDonald, & Joyce, 1997; Hickey et al., 1996). This is a simple apparatus consisting of five interlocking, colored, laminated circular disks that can be rotated over each other to form a type of pie chart. The disks, each a different color, are mounted centrally on a large backing disk that displays a 0–100 scale, from which the relative size of each segment can be measured. Following a structured interview to elicit the five cues, each of the five segments is labeled respectively with one of the five cues, using a different cue for each segment. The respondent adjusts the disks until the size of the segment corresponds to the relative importance (weight) of the cue. The disk can be adjusted until the respondent is satisfied that the final picture accurately reflects the relative importance of each area to his or her overall QOL. Although the method has the advantage of being simpler and faster to apply, its disadvantage, compared with the full method, is that it does not generate measures of internal reliability and validity. Using a similar method, normative data for a U.K. sample have recently been collected, and national population norms are available on pertinent domains of QOL, as are data on the relative importance of these domains to people with long-standing illness (Bowling, 1996).

Although the SEIQOL is an individually based measure, it can generate data that may be subjected to grouped analysis. The SEIQOL allows one to generate a global QOL score, the SEIQOL index score. This summary score is generated by multiplying each cue level by its respective weight and aggregating across the five cues. The Policy PC program (Executive Decision Services, 1986), which is used to derive the cue weights, also computes the R^2 statistic, which is a measure of the variance in overall QOL judgments explained by the combination of the five cues. This is an estimate of the internal validity of judgment analysis. The internal reliability may be calculated by correlating repeat case judgments. Therefore, the investigator can assess how well the particular judgment policy models the individual's assessment of QOL (R^2 and also how reliably the individual uses the policy (r).

SEIQOL and Response Shift

In the following sections of this chapter, we demonstrate, using data derived from a number of studies, the relevance of the SEIQOL to the measurement of response shift in adapting to cancer, aging, and dying. Figure 8.1 demonstrates how the various components of the SEIQOL might relate to the various types of response shift proposed by Schwartz and Sprangers (see chapters 1 and 6). If the SEIQOL were administered on two occasions, Time 1 and Time 2 (T1 and T2), changes in the content of the cues selected by respondents as being most important to their QOL would reflect reconceptualization. Changes in values would be reflected by changes in cue weights, whether these are derived by judgment analysis or by the direct weighting method. However, two complications arise here. First, the cues generated by the SEIQOL using the Policy PC program are relative cues and are constrained to sum to unity. Consequently, a change in one cue weight necessarily means that at least one of the other weights must change. Free weights that would be independent of each other may be more appropriate for determining changes in values. The second complication is that, in the full SEIQOL, cue weights are determined by using multiple regression analysis of data derived from visual analogue scales (VAS). QOL ratings are made on a horizontal VAS. Respondents first rate their current QOL and then judge the overall QOL that they would associate with a set of 30 profiles generated using their own cues. The levels of the cues in each profile are represented by means of a vertical VAS. A change in internal standards on either or both of these scales might result in a change in weights generated. Consequently, changes in weights might not be a pure indication of changes in values but might be influenced by changes in internal standards.

Schwartz and Sprangers have suggested that changes in internal standards might be assessed by having patients describe the relevant VAS anchors at T1 and T2. At T2, respondents could be asked to place their T1

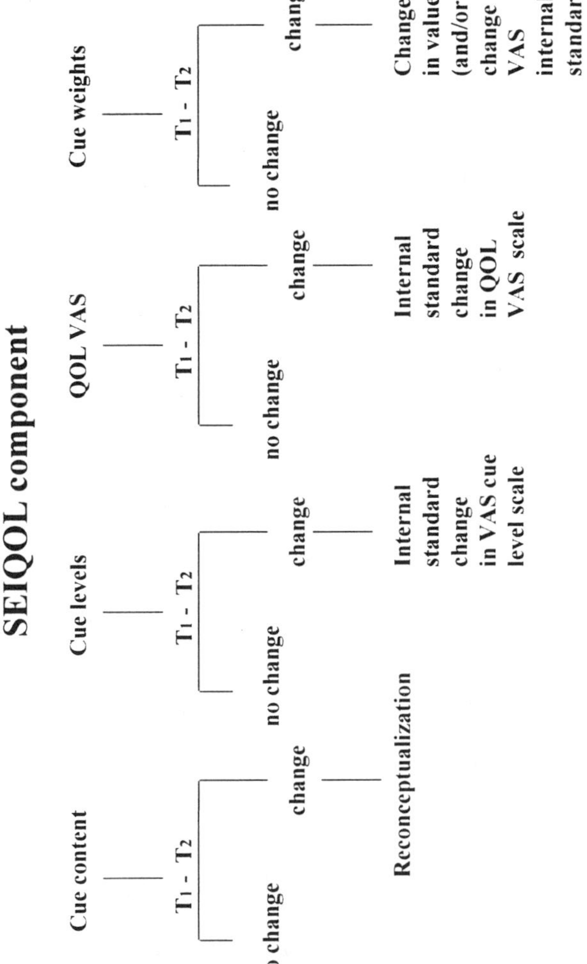

Figure 8.1. Application of the SEIQOL to the assessment of response shift.

anchors within the T2 anchored continuum. This would allow evaluation of the change in internal standards by making explicit change in anchors over time and in the relationship between anchors over time. An alternative approach would be to apply the thentest to both scales. At T2, the respondent would be asked to provide a renewed rating of their overall T1 QOL on the VAS and also to rate again their level of functioning in relation to each of the five cues nominated at T1 (for a critical discussion of the thentest approach, see chapter 10). These approaches may yet prove to be useful but, at present, a reliable and valid method of determining changes in internal standards using the SEIQOL has yet to be developed. Later sections of this chapter focus on the role of the SEIQOL in measuring reconceptualization and changes in values.

The type of data generated by the SEIQOL is illustrated in Figures 8.2, 8.3, and 8.4. Data are shown for a 51-year-old male patient who was terminally ill with prostate cancer with metastases in liver and bone (Waldron & O'Boyle, unpublished data). The SEIQOL was administered on three occasions, which retrospectively were found to coincide with eight, seven, and six months before his death. Figure 8.2 shows that the cues he selected were health, work, being pain free, family, and financial security. The levels show that he was doing reasonably well in relation to pain, family, and financial security and less well in the areas of health and work. The weights obtained by judgment analysis show that family was the most important cue, followed by health and being pain free. His SEIQOL index score was 61, and the combination of cues, weights, and levels, known as the judgment policy, had very high validity (R^2 = 0.89). He received radiotherapy for his pain between the first and second assessment and obtained good pain relief and improved energy for the fol-

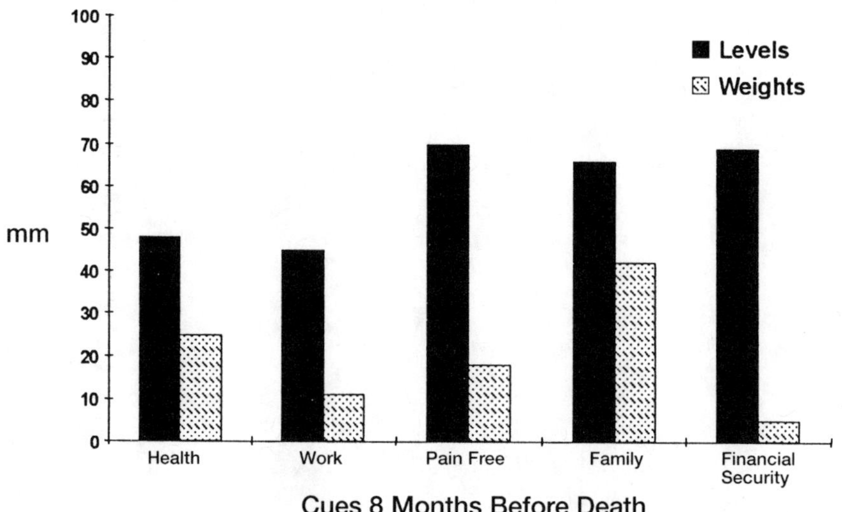

Figure 8.2. SEIQOL data for a 51-year-old male patient with advanced metastatic prostate cancer, obtained eight months before the patient died (SEIQOL index score = 61; R^2 = 0.89).

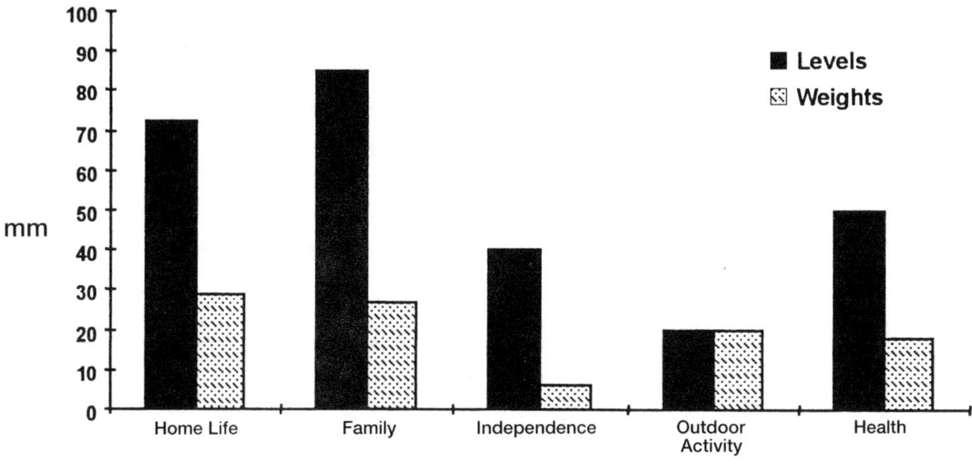

Figure 8.3. SEIQOL data for a 51-year-old male patient with advanced metastatic prostate cancer, obtained seven months before the patient died (SEIQOL index score = 59; R^2 = 0.93).

lowing three months. On the second assessment (see Figure 8.3), he chose home life, family, independence, outdoor activity, and health as the cues that were most important to his overall QOL. The SEIQOL index score was relatively unchanged at 59, and the validity of the judgment policy was again very high. The change in cues chosen represent a response shift characterized by reconceptualization and the change in the relative weights of the cues of family and health from the first to the second visits reflect response shifts characterized by changes in values. The patient was maintained on steroids between the second and third visits, his pain was

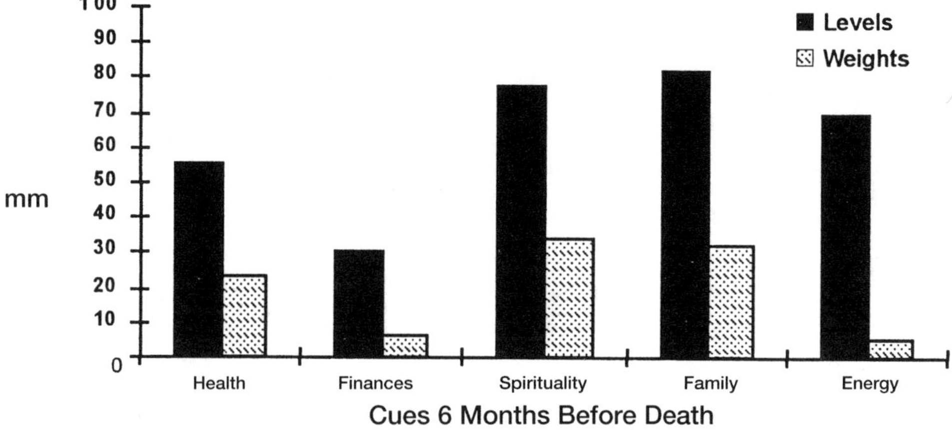

Figure 8.4. SEIQOL data for a 51-year-old male patient with advanced metastatic prostate cancer, obtained six months before the patient died (SEIQOL index score = 71; R^2 = 0.92).

well controlled, and he was generally feeling well, but he was increasingly aware that his condition was terminal. On the third visit (see Figure 8.4), he nominated health, finances, spirituality, family, and energy as the most important cues, with spiritual life now being rated as most important followed closely by family. His overall QOL actually improved, as is reflected in the SEIQOL score of 71, with high validity again being seen. This patient provides a good example of the dynamic nature of QOL with changes being seen in cues, levels, and weights over the course of three months.

Reconceptualization and Changes in Values

In one study, the SEIQOL was administered to a sample of 56 healthy elderly community residents on two occasions 12 months apart in order to determine the stability of cues, levels, and weights (Browne et al., 1994). As is shown in Table 8.1, relatively little change was seen in the nature of the cues selected over the study period. The only significant changes were in relation to finance, which was nominated more frequently at one year, and social and leisure activities, which were mentioned by fewer people at one year. Comparison of cues nominated at baseline and at one year revealed only one cue change on average (mean number of cue changes = 1.1; SD = 0.8; range = 0–3). Data on the stability of cues over time in healthy elderly individuals are also available from a study of hip replacement surgery in which a healthy control group was used (O'Boyle, McGee, Hickey, O'Malley, & Joyce, 1992). The SEIQOL method elicits five cues from each respondent at each application. As is shown in Table 8.2, the mean number of cue changes and the average changes in levels and weights were relatively modest over a 2-year period. These results indicate that the cues that older individuals judge to be important to their QOL remain relatively stable over periods as long as two years. The findings from these two studies suggest that, in the absence of a catalyst, recon-

Table 8.1. Cues Nominated by 56 Healthy Elderly People on the SEIQOL

Nominated cue	% of sample at baseline	% of sample at 1 year
Family/marriage	89	89
Social and leisure activities	95	59*
Health	91	87
Home/living conditions	80	89
Religion	75	84
Independence	16	14
Finance	25	43*
Friends/relationships	18	21
Work	5	7
Attitude to life/happiness	5	5

Note. SEIQOL = Schedule for the Evaluation of Individual Quality of Life. Data are from Browne et al., 1994. Adapted by permission. $*P < .05$ for X^2 comparisons.

Table 8.2. Changes in SEIQOL Cues, Levels, and Weights in a Sample of 20 Healthy Adults

	At 7.5 months			At 2 years		
SEIQOL data	M	SD	range	M	SD	range
Cue changes	1.1	0.94	0–3	1.3	0.83	0–3
Cue level changes	12.9	6.30	4–26	12.2	4.80	5–22
Cue weight changes	10.3	5.20	3.6–22.8	8.0	4.0	3.0–16.8

Note. SEIQOL = Schedule for the Evaluation of Individual Quality of Life. Age range 43–78 years; mean age 64. (O'Boyle, unpublished data)

ceptualization as indicated by cue changes, and changes in values as indicated by changes in cue weights, do not occur to any appreciable extent. This would support the proposal that response shifts in QOL require a catalyst (see chapter 1) and that, in the absence of such a catalyst, QOL is relatively stable over time.

Response Shift and Aging

In the study of healthy elderly people by Browne et al. (1994), a significant deterioration in health as measured by the symptoms of aging subscale of the Self-Evaluation of Life Function Scale was found (Table 8.3). This change in health did not result in a significant change in either overall QOL as measured by SEIQOL index scores or the relative weight assigned to health, for those who listed it as a SEIQOL cue. Given the deterioration in health seen in this group, one might have expected a response shift in relation to the value attached to health, but this did not occur. External observers often make judgments of patients' QOL that are at variance with those of the patient. One suspects that such judgments rely heavily on observed symptoms, and there is an implicit expectation that deterioration in health will necessarily result in the relative value of health increasing for the patient. In this study, such assumptions would have been unfounded, because the value of health did not increase despite its deterio-

Table 8.3. SEIQOL Index Scores, Symptom Levels, and Cue Weights for 56 Healthy Elderly People

	At baseline		At 1 year	
SEIQOL data	M	SD	M	SD
SEIQOL index (elderly)	82.1	12.2	80.1	11.2
Symptoms of aging	14.75	3.9	16.62	5.0**
Health cue weight	0.26	0.14	0.29	0.13

Note. SEIQOL = Schedule for the Evaluation of Individual Quality of Life. Age range 65–90 years; mean age 73.7. Data are from Browne et al., 1994. Adapted by permission. $^{**}P < .001$ for paired conversions between baseline and 1 year.

ration. Neither did QOL decrease. It follows that response shifts based on reconceptualization and changes in values should be measured directly from the patient and cannot be implied solely on the basis of external observations or by simply using objective measures of health that do not incorporate the unique perspective of the individual.

This and other SEIQOL data have shown that healthy elderly people select different cues in judging their QOL and rate their QOL as better than, or equal to, that of a younger sample. They did not show a deterioration in QOL or an increase in the relative importance of health, despite deterioration in health. These findings may be explained, at least in part, by response shifts associated with aging (O'Boyle, 1997).

One approach to understanding QOL in elderly people (Lundh & Nolan, 1996a, 1996b) has been to incorporate the model of aging proposed by Brandtstaedter and Greve (1994): Successful aging is seen as a dynamic process of balancing assimilative (maintaining current activities), accommodative (flexible goal adjustment), and immunizing (selective filtering) strategies in order to maintain a realistic and serviceable sense of self. The model of successful aging proposed by Baltes and Baltes and based on the Berlin Aging Study (Baltes & Baltes, 1990; Baltes, Mayer, Borchelt, Maas, & Wilms, 1996; Baltes, Mayer, Helmchen, & Thiessen, 1996), which focuses on the strategies for selection, optimization, and compensation, also has important implications for the study of QOL in elderly people. In particular, such theoretical models highlight the role of the adaptive nature of the aging person and make response shift a likely outcome of the developmental process. Using these strategies, individuals can contribute to their own successful aging. Although the biological nature of human aging limits more and more the overall range of possibilities in old age, the individual can adapt by selecting and concentrating on those domains that are of high priority and that involve convergence of environmental demands and individual motivations, skills, and biological capacity. Among the important implications of theoretical models such as these is the conclusion that any assessment of QOL in older people must concern itself with the unique concerns of individuals, their own subjective assessment of their circumstances, and the manner in which they adapt to and cope with change.

Response Shifts at the End of Life

The phenomenon of response shift has significant implications in situations where QOL judgments must be made well in advance of a medical intervention or where such an intervention is based on a proxy judgment of an individual's QOL. This is particularly relevant in the case of patients whose physical condition has deteriorated to a point where they are no longer capable of making decisions for themselves. It is generally accepted that patients have rights to have an input into decisions about their future, even when they are not capable of making decisions, and there is now considerable and growing interest in the development of advance directives or living wills. These require an individual to determine what course of action should be taken at some future point in time when their condition precludes them from making such a decision. Such judgments are based usually on a consideration of predicted symptoms and their impact on QOL. Advance directives are usually made when death or serious illness are abstract concepts and are likely to occur only in the distant future. The longitudinal validity of such directives is likely to be decreased if response shifts occur in patients' judgments over time. It seems likely that, if death becomes a more concrete threat, the patient's views may change and, should patients suddenly become unwell, the freedom to change the instruction may be removed (O'Boyle & Waldron, 1997; Potter, Stewart, & Duncan, 1994; Tsevat et al., 1998). We cannot assume that a decision made by patients while in good health or at a particular phase in their illness is necessarily representative of the decision they would make at a later stage when reconceptualization or changes in values are likely to have occurred.

One approach to the problems associated with advance directives has been to appoint a proxy or surrogate with the legal powers to make decisions on behalf of individuals who are not competent to do so themselves (O'Boyle, 1996). Proxy judgments are widely used, not only in relation to end-of-life decisions, but also in choosing appropriate care settings, deciding between alternative treatments, and judging the impact of treatments on patient symptomatology. The use of proxy judgments is based on the implicit assumption that a proxy can assume the values and preferences of the patient and furthermore that the proxy will be able to factor in any changes that might have occurred over time in the patient's views. Given the importance of such decisions, it is imperative to know how valid such proxy judgments are likely to be.

The SEIQOL–DW has recently been used to explore the discrepancy between proxy and respondent ratings of QOL (Browne, O'Boyle, & Coen, 2000). In a cross-sectional study, elderly couples ages 65 and older and married for at least five years were asked to rate their own QOL and to rate the QOL of their spouse, as the spouse would rate it. The study sample consisted of 21 healthy couples, 39 couples in whom one member was currently healthy and the other suffering from a chronic illness, and 20 couples in whom both were chronically ill. Findings showed that wives could accurately predict their husbands' judgments in all three conditions. Healthy husbands significantly underestimated their wives' ratings regardless of their level of health. In contrast, chronically ill husbands accurately rated the QOL of their chronically ill wives. Response shift provides one possible explanation for these findings in the case of the male partners. Although this was a cross-sectional study, it points to the conclusion that husbands who normally underestimate their wives' QOL can provide accurate judgments when they themselves have a chronic condition. It might be concluded that adapting to a disease causes a response shift that makes husbands more sensitive to similar adaptation in their wives. It is intriguing that wives were accurate regardless of their own or their husbands' condition.

Conclusion

The preceding examples illustrate instances in which some elements of response shift were measured using the SEIQOL. Although these studies did not specifically focus on response shift as a phenomenon, the SEIQOL does allow some aspects of response shift to be investigated. In particular, the method provides data that are relevant to changes in respondents' values and to reconceptualization. Further research is needed to develop measures of shifts in internal standards and to allow these to be separated from changes in values.

The philosophical and practical implications of response shift are likely to be significant. The occurrence of response shifts in QOL assessment provides support for the view that QOL is an individual dynamic phenomenon and that valid measures must incorporate the unique and changing perspective of the individual. Many of the studies that have used QOL as an outcome measure have not incorporated any assessment of response shift. Thus, the impact of conditions and their treatments on QOL may have been either underestimated or overestimated if, as seems likely, significant response shifts occurred. Because response shift is an important variable in judging QOL at the end of life, the phenomenon raises pertinent questions about the concurrent validity of proxy assessments and the predictive validity of advance directives.

References

Allison, P. J., Locker, D., & Feine, J. S. (1997). Quality of life: A dynamic construct. *Social Science and Medicine, 45*(2), 221–230.

Andrykowski, M. A., Brady, M. J., & Hunt, J. W. (1993). Positive psychosocial adjustment in potential bone marrow transplant recipients: Cancer as a psychosocial transition. *Psycho-Oncology, 2,* 261–276.

Baltes, M. M., Mayer, M., Borchelt, M., Maas, I., & Wilms, H. U. (1996). Everyday competence in old and very old age: An interdisciplinary perspective. *Ageing and Society, 13,* 657–680.

Baltes, P., & Baltes, M. (1990). Psychological perspectives on successful aging: The model of selective optimization with compensation. In P. Baltes & M. Baltes (Eds.), *Successful ageing: Perspectives from the behavioural sciences* (pp. 1–34). New York: Cambridge University Press.

Baltes, P., Mayer, K. M., Helmchen, H., & Thiessen, E. S. (1996). The Berlin Ageing Study (BASE): Overview and design. *Ageing and Society, 13,* 483–516.

Bennett, K. J., & Torrance, G. W. (1996). Measuring health state preferences and utilities: Rating scale, time trade-off and standard gamble techniques. In B. Spilke (Ed.), *Quality of life and pharmacoeconomics in clinical trials* (2nd ed., pp. 253–265). Philadelphia: Lippincott-Raven.

Bowling, A. (1996). The effects of illness on quality of life: Findings from a survey of households in Great Britain. *Journal of Epidemiology and Community Health, 50,* 149–155.

Brandstaedter, J., & Greve, W. (1994). The aging self: Stabilizing the protective process. *Developmental Review, 14,* 52–80.

Brehmer, B., & Joyce C. R. B. (Eds.). (1988). *Human judgment: The social judgment theory view*. Amsterdam: North-Holland.

Browne, J. P., O'Boyle, C. A., & Coen, R. F. (2000). *Assessment of quality of life in healthy and chronically ill older couples using an individual-centered approach*. Manuscript in preparation.

Browne, J. P., O'Boyle, C. A., McGee, H. M., Joyce, C. R. B., McDonald, N. J., O'Malley, K., & Hiltbrunner, B. (1994). Individual quality of life in the healthy elderly. *Quality of Life Research, 3,* 235–244.

Browne J. P., O'Boyle, C. A., McGee, H. M., McDonald, N. J., & Joyce, C. R. B. (1997). Development of a direct weighting procedure for quality of life domains. *Quality of Life Research, 6,* 301–309.

Brunswick, E. (1956). *Perception and the representative design of psychological experiments* (2nd ed.). Berkeley: University of California Press.

Cooksey, R. W. (1996). *Judgment analysis. Theory, methods and applications.* New York: Academic Press.

Dunbar, G. C., Stoker, M. J., Hodges, T. C. P., & Beaumont, G. (1992). The development of SBQuality of life—A unique scale for measuring quality of life. *British Journal of Medical Economics, 2,* 65–74.

Evans, R. W. (1991). Quality of life. *Lancet, 338,* 636.

Executive Decision Services. (1986). *Policy PC (Version 2.0) reference manual.* Albany, NY: Author.

Ferrans, C. E., & Powers M. J. (1995). Quality of life index: Development and psychometric properties. *American Journal of Nursing Science, 8,* 15–24.

Golembiewsky, R. T., Billingsley, K., & Yeager, S. (1976). Measuring change and persistence in human affairs: Types of change generated by OLD designs. *Journal of Applied Behavioural Research, 12,* 133–157.

Hammond, K. R., Stewart, T. R., Brehmer, B., & Steinmann, D. (1975). Social judgment theory. In M. F. Kaplan & S. Schwartz (Eds.), *Human judgment and decision processes: Formal and mathematical approaches.* New York: Academic Press.

Hickey, A. M., Bury, G., O'Boyle, C. A., Bradley, F., O'Reilly, F., & Shannon, W. (1996). A new short form individual quality of life measure (SEIQuality of life–DW): Applications in a cohort of individuals with HIV/AIDS. *British Medical Journal, 313,* 29–33.

Hunt, S. M. (1997). The problem of quality of life. *Quality of Life Research, 6,* 205–212.

Joyce, C. R. B., O'Boyle, C. A., & McGee, H. M. (Eds.). (1999). *Individual quality of life.* London: Harwood Academic Press.

Kreitler, S., Samario, C., Rapoport, Y., Kreitler, H., & Algor, R. (1993). Life satisfaction and health in cancer patients and healthy individuals. *Social Science and Medicine, 36*(4), 547–556.

Lundh, U., & Nolan, M. (1996a). Ageing and quality of life: 1. Towards a better understanding. *British Journal of Nursing, 5*(20), 1248–1251.

Lundh, U., & Nolan, M. (1996b). Ageing and quality of life: 2. Understanding successful aging. *British Journal of Nursing, 5*(21), 1291–1295.

O'Boyle, C. A. (1996). Quality of life in palliative care. In G. Ford & I. Lewin (Eds.), *Managing terminal illness* (pp. 37–47). London: RCP Publications.

O'Boyle, C. A. (1997). Measuring the quality of later life. *Philosophical Transactions of the Royal Society of London (B), 352,* 1871–1889.

O'Boyle, C. A., McGee, H. M., Hickey, A., Joyce, C. R. B., Browne, J., O'Malley, K., & Hiltbrunner, B. (1993). *The schedule for the evaluation of individual quality of life (SEI-Quality of life): Administration manual.* Dublin: Royal College of Surgeons in Ireland, Department of Psychology.

O'Boyle, C. A., McGee, H., Hickey, A., O'Malley, K., & Joyce, C. R. B. (1992). Individual quality of life in patients undergoing hip-replacement. *Lancet, 339,* 1088–1091.

O'Boyle, C. A., & Waldron, D. (1997). Quality of life issues in palliative medicine. *Journal of Neurology, 244,* S18–S25.

Potter, J. M., Stewart, D., & Duncan, G. (1994). Living wills: Would sick people change their minds? *Postgraduate Medical Journal, 70,* 818–820.

Ruta, D. A., Garratt, A. M., Leng, M., Russell, I. T., & McDonald, L. M. (1994). A new approach to the measurement of quality of life: The patient generated index. *Medical Care, 32,* 1109–1126.

Sprangers, M. A. G., & Aaronson, N. K. (1992). The role of health care providers and significant others in evaluating the quality of life of patients with chronic disease: A review. *Clinical Epidemiology, 45,* 743–760.

Stewart, T. R. (1988). Judgement analysis procedures. In B. Brehmer & C. R. B. Joyce (Eds.), *Human judgement: The social judgement theory* (pp. 41–74). Amsterdam: North Holland.

Thunedborg, K., Allerup, P., Bech, P., & Joyce, C. R. B. (1993). Development of the repertory grid for measurement of individual quality of life in clinical trials. *International Journal of Methods in Psychiatric Research, 3,* 45–56.

Tsevat, J., Dawson, N. V., Wu, A. W., Lynn, J., Soukup, J. R., Cook, E. F., Vidaillet, H., & Phillips, R. S. (1998). Health values of hospitalized patients 80 years or older. *Journal of the American Medical Association, 279*(5), 371–375.

9

Response Shift and Fatigue: The Use of the Thentest Approach

Mirjam A. G. Sprangers, Frits S. A. M. van Dam, Jenny Broersen, Litanja Lodder, Lidwina Wever, Mechteld R. M. Visser, Paul Oosterveld, and Ellen Smets

Self-reported symptoms and side effects have become increasingly important outcome parameters to evaluate the efficacy of both standard and experimental therapies for use with cancer patients. In clinical trials, the most simple design includes a pretreatment and posttreatment assessment. The assessment of symptoms in this pretest–posttest design (Campbell & Stanley, 1966) is based on the assumption that patients have a stable internalized standard of measurement for symptoms (Cronbach & Furby, 1970). This assumption may, however, be challenged. To the extent that cancer and its treatment induce symptoms and side effects and that patients learn to adapt to their increased symptom level, patients' internal standard of measurement may be changed (Andrykowski, Brady, & Hunt, 1993; Breetvelt & van Dam, 1991; Kagawa-Singer, 1993; Padilla et al., 1992).

This phenomenon is labeled *response shift* and is defined as a change in the meaning of one's self-evaluation of a target construct as a result of a change in the respondent's internal standards of measurement, a change in the respondent's values, or a reconceptualization of the target construct (see chapters 1 and 6). Although such shifting of internal criteria may help patients adapt to difficult circumstances, it may render pretest–posttest comparisons invalid. Because participants from a no-treatment or placebo control group do not undergo a treatment-induced response shift, posttest comparisons between experimental and control conditions are confounded

---

Adapted from "Revealing Response Shift in Longitudinal Research on Fatigue: The Use of the Thentest Approach," by M. A. G. Sprangers, F. S. A. M. van Dam, J. Broersen, L. Lodder, L. Wever, M. Visser, P. Oosterveld, and E. Smets, 1999, *Acta Oncologica, 38*, pp. 709–718. Copyright 1999 by Scandinavian University Press. Adapted with permission of Scandinavian University Press.

This chapter was supported by Dutch Cancer Society Grant NKI 90-A, awarded to Mirjam Sprangers.

We are indebted to Carolyn Schwartz for helpful discussions and comments on earlier drafts of this manuscript. This research was conducted while Mirjam Sprangers was on the staff of the Netherlands Cancer Institute.

as well. Response shift effects must be identified and measured for such comparisons to capture accurate and meaningful information. This chapter focuses on response shifts that result from changes in cancer patients' internal standards of assessing symptoms.

A Thentest Study of Cancer Patients

An attempt to measure response shift resulting from changes in internal standards of measurements has been made in the area of educational training interventions. Howard, Ralph, et al. (1979) recommended the extension of the conventional pretest–posttest design with a retrospective pretest, or "thentest." Although the thentest has been described in chapters 3 and 6, it will be described in more detail in this chapter. The procedure is as follows: At the posttest session, the participants fill out the self-report measure twice. First they are asked to report how they perceive themselves at present (conventional posttest), then they are asked to provide a renewed judgment about their pretreatment level of functioning (thentest). By taking the posttest and thentest in close proximity, it is assumed that these measures will be completed with respect to the same internal standard of measurement. Consequently, comparison of posttest and thentest scores would provide an unconfounded indication of the actual treatment effect. The comparison of the mean pretest and thentest scores would reflect an estimate of the magnitude and direction of response shift effects (see Figure 9.1).

The majority of studies that have included a thentest were performed in the area of educational training interventions. A considerable number of such studies indicated that the conventional pretest–posttest comparisons were affected adversely by response shift effects. The mean posttest minus thentest difference scores indicated a positive treatment effect, whereas results obtained by the conventional posttest minus pretest difference scores revealed no or minimal effects (Hoogstraten, 1982, 1985; Howard & Dailey, 1979; Howard, Dailey, & Gulanick, 1979; Howard, Schmeck, & Bray, 1979; Levinson, Gordon, & Skeff, 1990; Skeff, Stratos, & Bergen, 1992; Sprangers, 1989; Sprangers & Hoogstraten, 1987, 1989). Additionally, the posttest minus thentest difference scores were more in agreement with non-self-report measures of change than with conventional posttest minus pretest difference scores (Bray & Howard, 1980; Howard, Millham, Slaten, & O'Donnell, 1981; Howard, Ralph, et al., 1979; Skeff et al., 1992; Stieglitz, 1990). The accumulated results lend support to Howard's contention that, to the degree that a response shift occurs, inclusion of a thentest may provide not only an accurate estimate of the treatment effect, but also a sensitive assessment of participants' changes in internal standards.

The results found and the recommendations made with regard to the thentest pertain to the area of educational research. The question arises as to how the inclusion of a thentest may work in health-related research (Norman & Parker, 1996; see also chapter 3). We first used the thentest

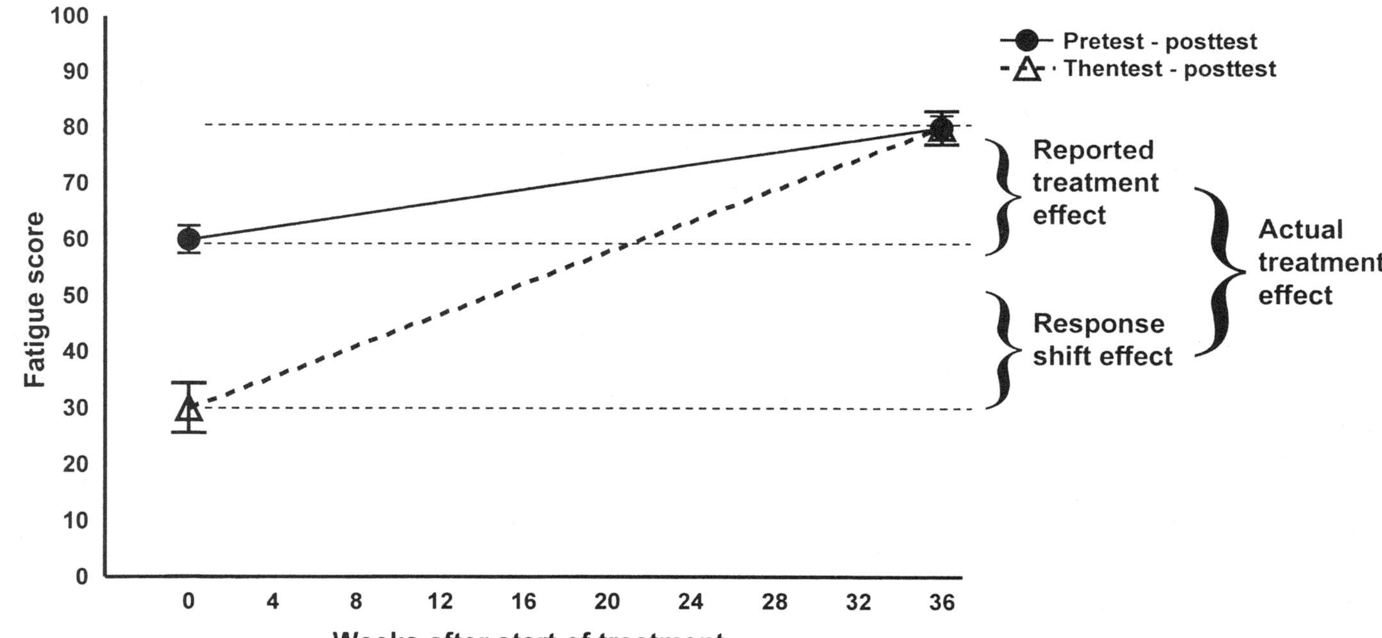

Figure 9.1. Example of results of the thentest approach to measuring response shifts in fatigue among cancer patients. Higher scores indicate higher levels of fatigue. Solid line indicates patients receiving treatment regimen 1, which does not affect fatigue level. Dotted line indicates patients receiving treatment regimen 2, which induces fatigue. Response shift effect = mean pretest minus thentest difference score. Actual treatment effect = mean posttest minus thentest difference score. Reported treatment effect = mean posttest minus pretest difference score.

in a pilot study with 26 outpatients receiving consecutive radiotherapy. These patients reported having become more tired as a result of radiotherapy and, as a consequence, minimized their fatigue level retrospectively (Sprangers, 1996; Sprangers & van Dam, 1994). We found these results sufficiently encouraging to replicate this study with a larger patient sample. The primary objective of the work reported in this chapter was to examine whether response shift occurred, resulting from changes in internal standards of measurement. Two hypotheses were formulated.

First, we expected, as in the pilot study, that patients whose fatigue levels increased, would retrospectively minimize their pretreatment symptom level, that is, have significantly lower mean thentest scores than mean pretest scores, with higher scores indicating a higher fatigue level (hypothesis 1). We also expected patients whose fatigue was alleviated to amplify retrospectively their pretreatment symptom level, that is, to have significantly higher mean thentest scores than mean pretest scores (hypothesis 2). Third, patients who have been tired for a relatively long period of time may have adapted their internal standards before entering the study. In such a case, a response shift is less likely to occur during the study period. We therefore expected that response shift would only occur in those patients whose fatigue started fairly recently. The third hypothesis thus specifies the length of the period prior to study entry during which patients reported to be tired. For exploratory reasons, we interviewed patients to examine whether they would provide verbalizations that would reflect response shift resulting from changes in internal standards of measurement.

Method

Sample selection. Newly diagnosed patients receiving consecutive radiotherapy for breast cancer subsequent to breast-conserving surgery and patients receiving primary radiotherapy of at least 13 fractions for lung or prostate cancer or for Hodgkin's lymphoma, respectively, were recruited from a cancer hospital in Amsterdam. The radiotherapy lasted between four weeks (lung cancer) and seven weeks (prostate cancer). All patients were ambulatory. To maximize the likelihood that we would evaluate patients from the beginning of the disease trajectory, we excluded patients who had cancer treatment previously, with the exception of those who had had breast-conserving surgery, or who had secondary tumors. Additionally, patients were excluded who lacked basic proficiency in Dutch or who were participating in concurrent quality-of-life (QOL) investigations. No restrictions were made with regard to age or performance status.

Dependent Measures

Fatigue. The European Organization for Research and Treatment of Cancer Core Quality of Life Questionnaire (EORTC QLQ-C30, version 1.0) was used (Aaronson et al., 1993). Given the focus of this chapter, only the results of the three-item fatigue scale will be reported. After completion of the EORTC QLQ-C30, patients were asked to indicate how long they had experienced fatigue if they had reported being tired during the past week (duration of fatigue). Answers were dichotomously scored (i.e., duration either shorter or longer than one month). The Multidimensional Fatigue Index (MFI-20) was also used, which includes subscales for general fatigue, physical fatigue, reduced activity, reduced motivation, and mental fatigue (Smets, Garssen, Cull, & de Haes, 1996). Higher scores on the QLQ-C30 and the MFI-20 indicate higher levels of fatigue.

Thentest. The instruction for the thentest begins with reviving patients' memory about the time they first completed the questionnaire, followed by the actual instruction: "I would like to ask you to provide a new judgment about the extent to which you had complaints at the time you first completed this questionnaire. Thus, I would like to ask you to complete the questionnaire as you now perceive yourself to have been during the week prior to your first session of radiotherapy." It was emphasized that patients were not asked to recall their responses but rather to provide a renewed judgment. Additionally, the items were adapted in such a way as to refer patients to the week prior to the first session.

Sociodemographic and clinical data. Sociodemographic data included age, gender, marital status, education, and employment. Clinical data included disease stage and nature and schedule of treatment, which were extracted from the patients' medical records. Patients were interviewed about their comorbidities.

Transition of fatigue. One question, based on the Subjective Significance Questionnaire (Osoba, Rodrigues, Myles, & Pater, 1995), inquired about the extent to which patients perceived to have changed with respect to fatigue since the week prior to the first session of radiotherapy. Patients rated their answers on a 7-point response scale ranging from 1 = a negative change to 7 = a positive change.

Interview. After introducing the interview topic (i.e., the responses to the pretest and the thentest), the interviewer asked patients to compare their answers to the posttest with those to the pretest. Permissible questions were whether the answers were generally in agreement or in disagreement as long as they were posed in this order. Interviewers were instructed to provide open, nonjudgmental probes (e.g., Can you amplify your answer? Can you give an example?). Interviewers were further instructed to elicit spontaneous or invited comparisons but not to use leading questions to address fatigue. The interviewers and the patients were blinded to the results of the pretreatment assessment.

Design and Procedures

The first assessment was carried out after the first session of radiotherapy and included the EORTC QLQ-C30, the question about the length of the period patients reported to be tired, the MFI-20, and the sociodemographic data, respectively. The second assessment took place after the last session of radiotherapy and included the administration of the EORTC QLQ-C30 and the MFI-20 as a conventional posttest and thentest, the interview, and subsequently the transition question on fatigue.

Statistical Analyses

Response shift. The transition score of fatigue was used to form mutually distinct patient subgroups, including patients who deteriorated and patients who improved over time. Deterioration or improvement was defined as a negative or positive change, respectively. The mean differences between the pretest and thentest scores of the fatigue scales were tested with one-tailed, dependent t tests (H_0: mean difference = 0). Data on stable patients are not reported in this chapter.

Length of period of symptoms and response shift. This hypothesis was examined in the subgroup of patients who (a) indicated having become more tired, by means of the transition score on fatigue, and (b) reported being tired less than one month at the time of the pretest (on the basis of the EORTC item: "Were you tired?"). One-tailed, dependent t tests were used to test for significant mean differences between the pretest and thentest scores. Given the exploratory nature of the current study, p values associated with chance probabilities less than .05 were considered statistically significant, despite the relatively large number of statistical tests. To examine the magnitude of these differences, effect sizes based on standardized differences between mean scores were calculated. Following Cohen (1988), effect sizes of .20, .50, and .80 were considered small, medium, and large, respectively.

Patients' verbalizations. The audiotaped interviews were transcribed by the interviewers and then rated by three researchers. Response shift was defined to be revealed when (1) patients report a difference between their responses to the pretest and thentest, which may either result from initial overrating or underrating, and (2) patients explicitly refer to a re-evaluation at the thentest of pretest levels of functioning. The transcribed interviews were rated independently in a fixed random order, that is, one researcher rated all interviews and two others each rated a random half. After discussion of each interview, consensus was achieved.

Results

Sample size. Of the 127 patients asked to participate in the study, 22 (17%) declined because of perceived lack of time or interest (n = 6), the study was perceived as emotionally too burdensome (n = 3), or other reasons (n = 13). The sociodemographic and clinical characteristics of the 105 participants at baseline are presented in Table 9.1.

Table 9.1. Baseline Sociodemographic and Clinical Characteristics of 105 Participants in a Thentest Study of Cancer Patients

Characteristic	n	%	Years
Age			
Median			63
Range			28–89
Gender			
Males	42	40	
Females	63	60	
Marital status			
Married	76	72	
Divorced	8	8	
Widowed	14	13	
Unmarried	7	7	
Education			
Compulsory only	80	76	
Advanced vocational	23	22	
University	2	2	
Employment			
Full-time	10	10	
Part-time	15	14	
Not employed	80	76	
Tumor			
Breast	59	56	
Lung	28	27	
Prostate	16	15	
Hodgkin's	2	2	
Disease stage			
Local	63	60	
Loco-regional	42	40	
Comorbidity			
Absent	25	24	

Response shift. Fifty-five patients reported becoming more tired. A systematic pattern of mean scores was not found. Because none of the mean thentest scores were significantly lower than the mean pretest scores, we rejected the first hypothesis (see Table 9.2). According to expectation, patients who became less tired (n = 13) had systematically higher mean thentest scores than mean pretest scores (hypothesis 2). With the exception of the mental fatigue scale of the MFI, the mean differences achieved statistical significance for all subscales, despite the small subsample sizes. Effect sizes of the significant differences were of a moderate to large magnitude (range: .58 to .94).

Length of period of symptoms and response shift. As expected, patients whose fatigue increased during radiotherapy and who reported being tired less than one month before study entry had lower mean thentest scores

Table 9.2. Mean Scores and Standard Deviations of the Pretest and the Thentest, Paired *t* Test Results, and Effect Sizes for Patients Who Reported Becoming More Tired or Less Tired Following Treatment

	More tired								Less tired							
	Pretest		Thentest						Pretest		Thentest					
Scale	*M*	*SD*	*M*	*SD*	*t*	df	*p*	d[3]	*M*	*SD*	*M*	*SD*	*t*	df	*p*	d[3]
MFI = 20[1]																
General Fatigue	10.62	3.99	10.96	3.94	−.66	49	.743	−.09	11.00	2.54	14.10	2.92	2.69	9	.008	.94
Physical Fatigue	9.40	3.96	10.48	3.91	−2.06	49	.978	−.29	9.40	2.90	12.90	3.35	2.50	9	.017	.79
Reduced Activity	11.34	3.56	11.10	4.78	.39	49	.349	.06	10.20	3.71	13.70	4.76	2.42	9	.020	.77
Reduced Motivation	10.10	4.31	11.62	4.70	−2.92	49	.997	−.41	8.90	3.41	12.40	6.20	1.84	9	.049	.58
Mental Fatigue	9.25	4.62	9.40	4.67	−0.25	47	.605	−.04	6.10	1.73	7.40	4.84	.88	9	.201	.28
EORTC QLQ = C30[2]																
Fatigue	25.25	18.58	22.83	18.20	1.05	54	.149	.14	30.77	10.30	37.61	14.73	2.31	12	.020	.64

Note. MFI = Multidimensional Fatigue Index. EORTC = European Organization for Research and Treatment of Cancer.
[1]The scale runs from 4 to 20, with higher values indicating a higher fatigue level.
[2]The scale runs from 0 to 100 (after linear transformation), with higher values indicating a higher fatigue level.
[3]Effect sizes are calculated according to the formula *M* (difference score)/*SD* (difference score) (Cohen, 1988). A positive effect size represents a result in accordance with the hypothesis.

than mean pretest scores in five of six subscales (see Table 9.3). Despite the small subsample size (n = 11), these differences achieved statistical significance for the general and mental fatigue scales of the MFI-20 and the fatigue scale of the EORTC QLQ-C30. The mean difference was marginally significant for the reduced activity scale of the MFI-20 (p = .056). In these cases, the effect sizes ranged from .53 to as high as 2.42.

Patients' verbalizations. Interviews were conducted with 74 patients (75%). The remaining 25 patients could not be interviewed primarily because of perceived lack of time (n = 9) or the unavailability of a quiet room (n = 9). When asked to compare their answers to the pretest and thentest, 5 patients were unable to make such comparisons. Additionally, 4 patients who claimed differences between their answers to the pretest and thentest gave comments that were found to be uncodable by the raters. These 9 interviews were excluded from the subsequent analyses of the interviews. The remaining 65 patients were articulate in documenting agreements or differences between their answers to the pretest and thentest.

Of the 14 patients who indicated that they perceived differences between their answers to the pretest and thentest, 11 clearly stated that some of their answers to the thentest provided a more favorable picture of their initial symptom level than their answers to the pretest. Interview excerpts referred to a reevaluation at the thentest of pretest levels of functioning. For example, a breast cancer patient stated that her response to the question about her fatigue was more positive at the thentest than at the pretest and explained,

> During the radiotherapy I became more tired. At that time, I may have thought that I was tired. But now I say no I was not tired at all. Now I am tired. . . . So, now I may look differently upon that week, while at that time I may have thought that I was dead tired.

Conversely, 6 patients (3 of whom also belong to the former category) indicated that some of the answers to the thentest provided a less favorable picture of their initial health status than their responses to the pretest (i.e., the category "initially better"). Again, interview excerpts were indicative of reevaluations of pretest levels of functioning. This is illustrated by the following example.

> When you are discharged from the hospital where you did not have any social activities . . . I think that I have thought at that time that it was improved. Now, when I look back I think it did not go that well, since I needed to do a lot of other things and I needed to rest and I had pain in my armpit.

Clearly, the majority of the patients (51) did not evidence response shift; they reported that their responses to the pretest and thentest were equivalent. As expected, most of these patients indicated that they were unchanged physically, as is illustrated by the following example: "My phys-

Table 9.3. Mean Scores and Standard Deviations of the Pretest and Thentest, Paired *t* Test Results, and Effect Sizes for Patients Who Became More Tired (Transition Score on Fatigue) and Who Reported to be Tired Less Than 1 Month Prior to Study Entry

	Pretest		Thentest					
Subscales	*M*	*SD*	*M*	*SD*	*t*	df	*p*	d[1]
MFI-20[2]								
General Fatigue	12.18	2.22	9.55	3.27	2.68	10	.012	.81
Physical Fatigue	10.45	4.11	9.18	3.37	1.01	10	.169	.30
Reduced Activity	11.27	2.24	9.27	4.29	1.75	10	.056	.53
Reduced Motivation	10.00	3.69	10.00	4.05	0.00	10	.500	0.00
Mental Fatigue	11.00	3.94	8.90	3.67	2.05	9	.036	.65
EORTC QLQ-C30[3]								
Fatigue	30.30	14.98	10.10	11.61	8.03	10	.000	2.42

Note. MFI-20 = Multidimensional Fatigue Index. EORTC QLQ-C30 = European Organization for Research and Treatment of Cancer Core Quality of Life Questionnaire, Version 1.0 (see p. 5).

[1]Effect sizes are calculated according to the following formula: *M* [difference score]/*SD* [difference score] (Cohen, 1988). A positive effect size represents a result in accordance with the hypothesis.

[2]The scale runs from 4 to 20, with higher values indicating a higher fatigue level.

[3]The scale runs from 0 to 100, with higher values indicating a higher fatigue level.

ical condition hasn't been changed by the radiotherapy . . . so there is not much shift in my perspective, in my judgement about then."

Interestingly, a number of comments referred to some of the underlying or mediating mechanisms of response shift (see chapter 1), including adaptation (e.g., "I think I look differently, more positive upon it than I did at that time . . . you get used to the fact that you have had cancer"), downward comparison (e.g., "Each day you see different people. This person has this, that one has that and then you compare yourself with them and then you think I am not doing that badly"), and the role of (unmet or overfulfilled) expectations (e.g., "Now it seems to be less severe, but now it is all past. In such a case you give an entirely different judgement than when you still have to face it").

Summary. There is evidence to suggest that cancer patients' internal standards for assessing their level of fatigue is not stable. In this chapter we have used the thentest approach to detect such response shift effects in self-report fatigue measures. The pattern of mean scores indicative of response shift effects was found in two subsamples of patients, despite the small subsample sizes: (1) those who became less tired and (2) those who reported having become tired as a result of radiotherapy and whose fatigue started shortly before study entry. The majority of patients reported in interviews that their responses to the pretest and thentest were equivalent. Those who thought their responses were dissimilar indicated that their answers to the thentest provided either a more or less favorable picture of their pretreatment level of fatigue. Verbalizations to justify these responses were found to be indicative of response shift resulting from changes in internal standards. It is thus likely that response shift resulting from changes in internal standards of measurement occurred in two distinct patient subgroups: patients experiencing diminishing levels of fatigue and patients facing early stages of adaptation to increased levels of fatigue.

Design Limitations

A number of limitations of the current study merit attention. First, a considerable number of patients remained stable over time with respect to reported fatigue ($n = 31$). Consequently, the selection of the patient sample (local or locoregional disease), the choice of the intervention (i.e., radiotherapy with curative intent), and the time lag between pretest and thentest (four to seven weeks) may have been insufficient in capturing the change in health status needed for response shift effects to occur, at least in a considerable number of patients. Second, criterion measures of change that would allow validation of the current approach were not included. Third, the transition score on fatigue may be criticized for its self-reported nature. Such assessments are subject to various sources of reporting error, such as recall bias and cognitive dissonance (Aseltine, Carlson, Fowler, &

Barry, 1995). We therefore used this measure only as a stratification and not as a criterion variable. Finally, forming two extreme groups (i.e, those who become more or less tired), although inherent to the testing of response shift, may induce regression-to-the-mean effects. However, the pronounced results of the patients who become less tired and of those whose fatigue started recently appear to refute this alternative explanation. Clearly, there is need for additional research to replicate and test the validity of our findings.

Two general remarks are in order. First, to avoid a misunderstanding of the implications of this study, we are not recommending that a thentest be used as a substitute for a pretest. A pretest is an indispensable part of the research design because, in addition to the thentest, it allows for assessing the amount and direction of response shift effects. Second, although the thentest approach was designed to assess change in internal standards of measurement, it is difficult to imagine that this change would occur without affecting the conceptualization of the construct. If new experiences will expand (or contract) the response scale, then the anchors and the intervals will have different meaning. Thus, change in conceptualization of the target construct may be implied by the thentest approach (see also chapter 6).

Implications for Future Research

The thentest approach itself needs to be subject to rigorous testing in future research. Studies are needed to examine the extent to which the thentest is a feasible and useful method for assessing response shift effects in the context of clinical trials or other longitudinal designs. For example, given the relative cognitive complexity of the task, future research needs to examine the extent to which completion of the thentest on a routine basis is feasible. A further question is related to the extent to which the thentest can be used with three or more assessment points and how data derived from such complex designs need to be analyzed statistically. Additionally, the extent to which the thentest is an appropriate measure for assessing physical symptoms needs to be further examined. For example, a certain level of prevalence of symptoms at the pretest is required for detecting response shift effects. When the prevalence is low at the pretest —indicating that patients do not have this symptom—patients cannot retrospectively adjust the responses to a lower symptom level. A response shift resulting from retrospective minimization of the pretreatment level is then problematic. This could point to an area where such response shift effects are less likely to occur or, alternatively, to a limitation in the usefulness of the thentest.

Second and most critically, research is needed that examines the extent to which a thentest is a valid instrument in capturing response shift effects in the context of health-related research. Thentests, like all self-report measures, are susceptible to confounding effects, such as cognitive dissonance, social desirability, response-style effects, and recall bias. For example, if patients undergo a medical or psychosocial intervention intended to improve their health condition, participants may feel inclined to adjust retrospectively their initial level of functioning to report improvement in order to justify their invested effort (cognitive dissonance) or to please the clinician (social desirability), which in turn may induce selective recall (recall bias). We are still uncertain about the extent to which these potential contaminants may be operative in health-related research. The viability of such alternative explanations might be tested by experimental techniques.

For example, by including a placebo control condition, the potential confounding influence of cognitive dissonance and social desirability can be examined (Sprangers & Hoogstraten, 1991). Response-style effects may be introduced by the administration procedure where the thentest is being made dependent on the posttest. Alternative administration procedures may be tested to examine the robustness of the thentest to such manipulations. For example, the order of the posttest and thentest may be reversed (Sprangers & Hoogstraten, 1989; Terborg & Davis, 1982), or respondents may complete the thentest in conjunction with their own pretest data (Guyatt, Berman, Townsend, & Taylor, 1985). With respect to the potential influence of recall bias, future research should address the optimal time interval for accurate thentest measurement, and the degree of salience needed for the conditions that are to be reevaluated from a potentially recalibrated standard of measurement.

An important question that remains is, by means of what kind of methodology can response shift be distinguished from recall bias (Collins, Graham, Hansen, & Johnson, 1985; Howard, Dailey, & Gulanick, 1979; Mancuso & Charlson, 1995)? One way to proceed is to include a memory test of participants' initial responses, to examine the concordance among the responses to the memory test, baseline assessment, and thentest (Collins et al., 1985; Howard, Dailey, & Gulanick, 1979). Finally, given the limitations inherent in any single measurement approach, studies are needed to detect and examine alternative approaches to detecting response shifts resulting from changes in internal standards of measurement as well as from changes in values and conceptualization (see chapter 6).

Such studies are needed to provide us with the insight into the extent to which the thentest and other measurement strategies are useful and valid for assessing the amount and direction of response shifts in health-related research. Such research is of paramount importance for treatment evaluations, especially insofar as response shifts may jeopardize estimates of treatment effects as patients adapt to treatment toxicities or disease progression over time or, alternatively, to improvements in their health. Response shifts may thus reduce the usefulness of self-reported outcomes in the context of clinical trials or other longitudinal research if these shifts are not explicitly measured. By assessing response shifts, changes in perceived symptoms and functioning over time will be assessed more validly and sensitively.

References

Aaronson, N. K., Ahmedzai, S., Bergman, B., Bullinger, M., Cull, A., Duez, N. J., Filiberti, A., Flechtner, S., Fleishman, S. B., de Haes, J. C. J. M., Kaasa, S., Klee, M., Osoba, D., Razavi, D., Rofe, P. B., Schraub, S., Sneeuw, K., Sullivan, M., & Takeda, F. (1993). The European Organization for Research and Treatment of Cancer QLQ-C30: A quality-of-life instrument for use in international clinical trials in oncology. *Journal of the National Cancer Institute, 85*, 365–376.

Andrykowski, M. A., Brady, M. J., & Hunt, J. W. (1993). Positive psychosocial adjustment in potential bone marrow transplant recipients: Cancer as a psychosocial transition. *Psycho-Oncology, 2*, 261–276.

Aseltine, R. H., Carlson, K. J., Fowler, F. J., & Barry, M. J. (1995). Comparing prospective and retrospective measures of treatment outcomes. *Medical Care, 33*, AS67–AS76.

Bray, J. H., & Howard, G. S. (1980). Methodological considerations in the evaluation of a teacher-training program. *Journal of Educational Psychology, 72*, 62–70.

Breetvelt, I. S., & van Dam, F. S. A. M. (1991). Underreporting by cancer patients: The case of response shift. *Social Science & Medicine, 32*, 981–987.

Campbell, D. T., & Stanley, J. C. (1966). *Experimental and quasi-experimental designs for research*. Chicago: Rand McNally.

Cohen, J. (1988). *Statistical power analysis for the behavioral sciences*. Hillsdale, NJ: Lawrence Erlbaum Associates.

Collins, L. M., Graham, J. W., Hansen, W. B., & Johnson, A. C. (1985). Agreement between retrospective accounts of substance use and earlier reported substance use. *Applied Psychological Measurement, 9*, 301–309.

Cronbach, L. J., & Furby, L. (1970). How we should measure "change"—or should we? *Psychological Bulletin, 74*, 68–80.

Guyatt, G. H., Berman, L. B., Townsend, M., & Taylor, D. W. (1985). Should study subjects see their previous responses? *Journal of Chronic Disease, 38*, 1003–1007.

Hoogstraten, J. (1982). The retrospective pretest in an educational training context. *Journal of Experimental Education, 50*, 200–204.

Hoogstraten, J. (1985). Influence of objective measures on self-reports in a retrospective pretest–posttest design. *Journal of Experimental Education, 53*, 207–210.

Howard, G. S., & Dailey, P. R. (1979). Response shift bias: A source of contamination of self-report measures. *Journal of Applied Psychology, 64*, 144–150.

Howard, G. S., Dailey, P. R., & Gulanick, N. A. (1979). The feasibility of informed pretests in attenuating response-shift bias. *Applied Psychological Measurement, 3*, 481–494.

Howard, G. S., Millham, J., Slaten, S., & O'Donnell, L. (1981). Influence of subject response style effects on retrospective measures. *Applied Psychological Measurement, 5*, 89–100.

Howard, G. S., Ralph, K. M., Gulanick, N. A., Maxwell, S. E., Nance, S. W., & Gerber, S. K. (1979). Internal invalidity in pretest–posttest self-report evaluations and a re-evaluation of retrospective pretests. *Applied Psychological Measurement, 3*, 1–23.

Howard, G. S., Schmeck, R. R., & Bray, J. H. (1979). Internal invalidity in studies employing self-report instruments: A suggested remedy. *Journal of Educational Measurement, 16*, 129–135.

Kagawa-Singer, M. (1993). Redefining health: Living with cancer. *Social Science & Medicine, 37*, 295–304.

Levinson, W., Gordon, G., & Skeff, K. (1990). Retrospective versus actual pre-course self-assessments. *Evaluation Health Profession, 13*, 445–452.

Mancuso, C. A., & Charlson, M. E. (1995). Does recollection error threaten the validity of cross-sectional studies of effectiveness? *Medical Care, 33*, AS77–AS88.

Norman, P., & Parker, S. (1996). The interpretation of change in verbal reports: Implications for health psychology. *Psychology Health, 11*, 301–314.

Osoba, D., Rodrigues, G., Myles, J., & Pater, J. (1995). Significance of changes in health-related quality of life (QOL) scores in women receiving chemotherapy for recurrent or metastatic breast cancer. *Quality of Life Research, 4*, 468–469.

Padilla, G. V., Grant, M. M., Lipsett, J., Anderson, P. R., Rhiner, M., & Bogen, C. (1992). Health quality of life and colorectal cancer. *Cancer, S70*, 1450–1456.

Skeff, K. M., Stratos, G. A., & Bergen, M. R. (1992). Evaluation of a medical faculty development program. *Evaluation Health Profession, 15*, 350–366.

Smets, E. M. A., Garssen, B., Cull, A., & de Haes, J. C. J. M. (1996). Application of the Multidimensional Fatigue Inventory (MFI-20) in cancer patients receiving radiotherapy. *British Journal of Cancer, 73*, 242–245.

Sprangers, M. (1989). Response-shift bias in program evaluation. *Impact Assessment Bulletin, 7*, 153–166.

Sprangers, M. A. G. (1996). Response shift bias: A challenge to the assessment of patients' quality of life in cancer clinical trials. *Cancer Treatment Reviews, 22SA*, 55–62.

Sprangers M., & Hoogstraten, J. (1987). Response-style effects, response-shift bias and a bogus-pipeline. *Psychological Reports, 61*, 579–585.

Sprangers, M., & Hoogstraten, J. (1989). Pretesting effects in retrospective pretest–posttest designs. *Journal of Applied Psychology, 74*, 265–272.

Sprangers, M., & Hoogstraten, J. (1991). Subject bias in three self-report measures of change. *Methodika, 5*, 1–13.

Sprangers, M. A. G., & van Dam, F. S. A. M. (1994). *Response-shift bias in longitudinal quality of life research: A first, exploratory study* [Report]. Amsterdam: The Netherlands Cancer Institute.

Stieglitz, R. D. (1990). Validätsstudien zum retrospetkiven Vortest in der Therapieforschung. *Zeitschrift für Klinische Psychologie, 19*, S144–150.

Terborg, J. R., & Davis, G. A. (1982). Evaluation of a new method for assessing change to planned job redesign as applied to Hackman and Oldham's job characteristic model. *Organizational Behavior and Human Performance, 28*, 112–128.

10

Discussion: Methodological Pathways

Mirjam A. G. Sprangers and Carolyn E. Schwartz

Investigating and testing the methods presented in this section of the book are the key to beginning to integrate response shift into health-related quality-of-life (QOL) research. The field of response shift challenges us to rethink the assumptions underlying current methods of assessing change. It highlights the dynamic nature of QOL by emphasizing that static, cross-sectional assessments of different patients at various points in the disease trajectory do not adequately reflect the experience of an individual over the entire disease trajectory. At this time, however, the questions arising from this construct far outnumber its canons. The purpose of this integrative discussion is to highlight the conundrums facing this emerging area of investigation.

In the first chapter of this section (chapter 6), we present a host of methods for assessing response shift, some involving primary data collection and others utilizing more recent quantitative techniques. We also recommend a reexamination of some of the tenets of psychometric theory. Empirical data from subsequent chapters illustrate a number of the suggested methods. In chapter 7, Llewellyn-Thomas and Schwartz provide guidelines to distinguish response shift from systematic biases when studying patients' preferences for different health states. O'Boyle, McGee, and Browne (chapter 8) focus on the Schedule for Evaluation of Individual Quality of Life (SEIQOL) as an example of an individualized measure. In chapter 9, Sprangers et al. exemplify the use of the thentest as a design approach for assessing response shift. Thus, each chapter contributes to an understanding of the methodological pathways to assess response shift or exemplifies some of the available tools for examining response shift in QOL data. It should be noted that chapters 2, 3, 4, 12, 13, and 14 also include quantitative or qualitative data on response shift, as revealed by primary or secondary analysis.

In the chapters containing empirical data, examples are provided of qualitative, design-, and preference-based methods. The majority of these measures are relatively new, including the goal-change approach of Rapkin (chapter 4), the SEIQOL presented by O'Boyle et al. (chapter 8), and

This chapter was funded in part by Agency for Health Care Policy and Research Grant 1 RO1 HSO 8582-03 to Carolyn Schwartz.

We thank Rebecca Gelman for helpful discussions.

preference-based mapping illustrated by Lenert et al. (chapter 14). Conversely, the thentest approach presented in chapter 9 has a long history in addressing changes in internal standards, which has an early foundation in educational research (Howard et al., 1979). Moreover, the thentest is relatively easy to apply, because it requires the administration of an extra questionnaire or, alternatively, a selection of items, with a thentest instruction. It is therefore tempting to incorporate the thentest routinely in ongoing research to measure changes in internal standards.

However, a cautionary note is in order. Self-report measures are susceptible to contaminating effects, such as mood, social desirability, cognitive dissonance, and response-style effects. The inclusion of retrospection is expected to exacerbate these biases (Howard et al., 1979). Whereas studies of educational training interventions indicate that the thentest is equally or even less vulnerable to such contaminants than is the conventional pretest (Howard, Millham, Slaten, & O'Donnell, 1981; Sprangers, 1988; Sprangers & Hoogstraten, 1987), we do not yet know the extent to which these potential confounders are operant in health-related psychosocial research. Additionally, the potential influence of recall bias in thentest ratings merits close attention. Because these potential validity threats to the thentest are by no means trivial, they warrant thorough evaluation. Suggestions for such validation studies are provided in chapter 9.

Establishing Validity and Reliability

A critical issue regarding all the methods to detect response shift is that the phenomenon of interest, response shift, and these methods are interrelated. If no evidence of response shift effect is found, this may either allude to the genuine absence of a response shift effect or to the inadequacy of the methods in detecting such an effect. Similarly, positive results may be attributable to the existence of response shift effect only to the extent that the measurement strategy used is valid. It is difficult to circumvent this circularity other than to test the various methods rigorously by formulating explicit hypotheses and by including criterion measures of change, that is, objective assessments of health status.

Another recommendation is to examine the convergent validity of these approaches. This procedure involves triangulating methods assessing the same component of response shift to determine the extent to which their results point in the same direction. By thus examining their convergent validity, methods can be identified that are not valid or sensitive enough to detect response shift. This procedure is strengthened by the inclusion of the above-mentioned criterion measures of change. Similarly, it is unclear whether methods addressing different components of response shift should be expected to point in the same direction. For example, if a measure of changes in internal standards suggests a response shift, then should measures assessing changes in values and conceptualization also suggest a response shift? If they do not, does that suggest that one or more of the methods is not valid or not sensitive enough? Convergent validity, thus, presents a particular challenge to this line of investigation.

Another step in establishing the validity of the response shift methods would be to identify an appropriate control group. This step, however, is less than straightforward, because both health state changes and time in itself are hypothesized to constitute catalysts of response shift. An alternative strategy might be to identify comparison groups that would be expected to engage in different directions or types of response shift. People who would be expected to engage in different directions of response shift would be people whose health state either deteriorates or improves. In the former case, one might expect them to lower their internal standards, shift their values to nonhealth domains, and reconceptualize QOL in terms of interpersonal factors instead of focusing on professional accomplishments. Conversely, patients whose health state improves might raise their internal standards, shift their values increasingly to health-related domains, and reconceptualize QOL in terms of physical role performance. As is noted in the theoretical discussion of this book, patients with stable health might not be expected to engage in response shifts. The impact of time might, however, be a catalyst of response shift such that people adapt to health state changes with the passage of time. These gaps in our knowledge of relevant parameters for catalysts of response shift suggest that there is a need for carefully planned research to document response shifts in patients with different disease trajectories, with an eye toward identifying whether including a medically ill control group is feasible.

Another critical issue concerns the interdependence of measures. If multiple antecedents and mechanisms are being assessed simultaneously to test, for example, the theoretical models of Sprangers and Schwartz or of Lepore and Eton, then analytic complications arise that need to be addressed. For example, personality characteristics such as those considered antecedents of response shift (e.g., optimism, mastery, and self-esteem), are likely to be highly intercorrelated, leading to the statistical problem of multicollinearity. Although this problem can be partially solved by selecting the measure that shares the most variance with the other measures, one would end up dropping a number of measures from the analysis, resulting in a wasted data collection effort. Similar problems may arise when assessing multiple putative mechanisms of response shift (e.g., reframing expectations, reordering goals, initiating social comparisons), all of which may be interconnected, and thus multicollinear to some extent. One possible solution to this type of problem is to plan studies with adequate sample sizes (i.e., 200 participants) to allow structural equation modeling, a statistical method that can accommodate the complexity involved in interdependence.

A final albeit obvious consideration is to evaluate the reliability of the various methods of response shift. Test–retest reliability should be assessed for self-report measures and of the change scores. For questionnaires with a multiple-item structure, internal consistency reliability also needs to be examined. For a hierarchically ordered measure, item-response theory approaches could be applied to assess the consistency of the response pattern.

All of these issues of validity and reliability need to be taken into account to further this line of research. The potentially tautological caveats involved in rigorously addressing validity and reliability of response shift measures will require careful thinking, innovative approaches to validating the measures of response shift, and a strong reliance on theory-driven research. The chapters included in this section of the book provide an initial guide to conducting such response shift investigations. They also point to the areas where the methodological approaches require further development and refinement. Despite their initial stage, these developments provide an invitation to examine response shift in upcoming studies. It is also possible, however, to infer response shift phenomena in existing data. The next section of the book will explore how reexamining existing data from a response shift perspective may lead to an intriguing interpretation of the findings.

References

Howard, G. S., Millham, J., Slaten, S., & O'Donnell, L. (1981). Influence of subject response style effects on retrospective measures. *Applied Psychological Measurement, 5,* 89–100.

Howard, G. S., Ralph, K. M., Gulanick, N. A., Maxwell, S. E., Nance, S. W., & Gerber, S. K. (1979). Internal invalidity in pretest-posttest self-report evaluations and a re-evaluation of retrospective pretests. *Applied Psychological Measurement, 3,* 1–23.

Sprangers, M. (1988). *Response shift and the retrospective pretest: On the usefulness of retrospective pretest-posttest designs in detecting training related response shifts.* Gravenhage, The Netherlands: Het Instituut voor Onderzoek van het Onderwijs S.V.O.

Sprangers M., & Hoogstraten, J. (1987). Response-style effects, response-shift bias and a bogus-pipeline. *Psychological Reports, 61,* 579–585.

Part III

New Perspectives on Existing Data

11

Clinical Understanding and Clinical Implications of Response Shift

Ira B. Wilson

. . . for there is nothing either good or bad but thinking makes it so.
–*Hamlet*, Act 2, Scene 2

The mind is in its own place, and it itself
Can make a heaven of hell, a hell of heaven.
–John Milton, *Paradise Lost*, Book 1

In this chapter I discuss the clinical implications of response shift. I have three principal goals: (a) to describe response shift in a clinical setting; (b) to show how response shift can help shed some light on several difficult problems in clinical medicine, specifically somatization and hypochondriasis, and placebo effects; and (c) to discuss aspects of the role of response shift in clinical care, specifically its implications for physician–patient communication and its relationship to the phenomenon of use of complementary and alternative medical therapies. Another goal of this discussion is to help clinical scientists better understand the arguments about response shift that are made by social scientists, health psychologists, and researchers in organizational behavior.

The phenomenon of response shift can occur in any field in which self-report data are collected. Clinicians may not consider clinical medicine a discipline characterized by self-report data, but much of the physician–patient interaction consists of talk (Roter & Hall, 1992), and the medical history is a critical component of the diagnostic process. The physician–patient relationship, physician–patient communication, and interpersonal care are all increasingly the subject of study, particularly as data have emerged that better communication and better interpersonal care can translate not only into more patient satisfaction but also into improved

Adapted from "Clinical Understanding and Clinical Implications of Response Shift," by I. B. Wilson, 1999, *Social Science & Medicine, 48*(11), pp. 1577–1588.

This work was supported in part by a Picker Commonwealth Scholars Award and a Robert Wood Johnson Generalist Faculty Scholars Award to Ira Wilson.

health outcomes (Greenfield, Kaplan, & Ware, 1985; Greenfield, Kaplan, Ware, Yano, & Frank, 1988).

The focus in this chapter will be on response shifts that are related to quality of life (QOL) in clinical care. *Response shift*, as the term will be used here, refers to a change in the meaning of one's self evaluation of a target construct as a result of (a) a change in the respondent's internal standards of measurement, or scale recalibration; (b) a change in the respondent's values, or the importance of component domains constituting the target construct; or (c) a reconceptualization of the target construct (see chapters 1 and 6).

Organizational psychologists interested in the methodological challenges of measuring changes in individuals' reports about their beliefs and attitudes have developed a typology that posits three types of change: (a) alpha change, referring to "true" behavioral change; (b) beta change, referring to scale recalibration; and (c) gamma change, referring to reconceptualization (Armenakis, 1988). Norman and Parker (1996) have discussed true behavioral change, scale recalibration, and concept redefinition in the context of a stress management intervention. True behavioral change occurs when an individual learns new coping strategies, applies them, and reports less stress after the intervention. To understand scale recalibration, imagine a woman who reports moderate stress when surveyed prior to the intervention. During the intervention, she realizes that she was under more stress than she had previously appreciated; when surveyed after the intervention, she reports more stress than before. In this case there is not more stress in her life after the intervention, but the intervention caused her to assess differently the amount of stress she experienced; the scale used to report stress has been recalibrated. To understand concept redefinition, imagine a man who thinks about stress as something acute and usually related to deadlines at work. When surveyed prior to the intervention, he responds with this framework in mind. During the intervention he learns that there are different kinds of stress, including acute stress, chronic stress, daily hassles, positive stress, and negative stress; subsequently he reconceptualizes his stress. When he responds to the postintervention survey, he uses this much broader framework and reports a higher level of stress than before—not because anything has changed in his life, but because stress has a different meaning to him than previously. For any such intervention, a person could in theory experience any or all of these types of change.

Investigators interested in the impact of interventions on the behaviors of individuals or organizations want to prove that true behavioral change has occurred. This requires that scale recalibration and concept redefinition be measured and adjusted for, if present. Clinicians have not generally thought about changes in health using this vocabulary. However clinicians, researchers, and patients are increasingly interested in understanding and measuring QOL (Guyatt, Feeny, & Patrick, 1993; Testa & Simonson, 1996). QOL considerations are particularly important in the treatment of chronic conditions such as hypertension (Testa, Anderson, Nackley, & Hollenberg, 1993), diabetes (Jacobson, Cleary, & Baker, 1996), arthritis (Bradley, Brandt, Katz, Kalasinski, & Ryan, 1991), HIV infection (Lenderking, Gelber, Cotton, Cole, & Goldhirsch, 1994), and cancer (Ganz, 1994), which often require long-term adherence to complex and potentially toxic treatment regimens. In clinical medicine, response shift is often much more than a methodological complication to be identified, measured, and controlled for—it is sometimes one of the primary objectives of clinical care.

Decomposition of Response Shift

Response shift is a complex phenomenon. Part of the goal of this chapter is to make response shift more concrete by relating it to clinical phenomena familiar to and understood by physicians and patients. I start by trying to decompose and further define response shift. The notion of response shift contains within it two important concepts: response and shift. The concept of *response* refers to the fact that patients make an assessment, judgment, report, or rating of a health state. The notion of *shift* implies a change in the patient's response.

What Is the Clinical Meaning of Response?

Earlier I stated that the focus in this chapter would be on QOL in clinical care. In previous work, Cleary and I (Wilson & Cleary, 1995) developed a conceptual framework for clinical outcomes that is useful in understanding the concepts of response and response shift as they are used here. The model posits causal linkages between five types of outcome measures: biological or physiological variables, symptoms, functioning, general health perceptions, and overall QOL (see Figure 11.1). Biological or physiological variables are variables that assess the function of cells and organs; examples are blood glucose, serum cholesterol, or blood pressure. Such biological and physiological variables are usually assessed by instruments, not by self-report. Symptoms are patients' perceptions of an abnormal physical or psychological state; they are by definition subjective.

Functioning refers to assessments of ability to perform specific tasks or functions. There are different kinds of functioning, such as physical functioning, social functioning, emotional functioning, and role functioning. These are usually patients' assessments, but functioning can also be observed and reported by others. General health perceptions are patients' global perceptions about their health and take account of the weights or values that patients attach to different symptoms or functional impairments. Finally, overall QOL is a measure of life satisfaction that may have little or nothing to do with health. For example, overall QOL may be strongly influenced by factors such as an individual's economic and employment status, his or her family situation, or the political environment. Because this is a discussion of medical care, the term *health-related qual-*

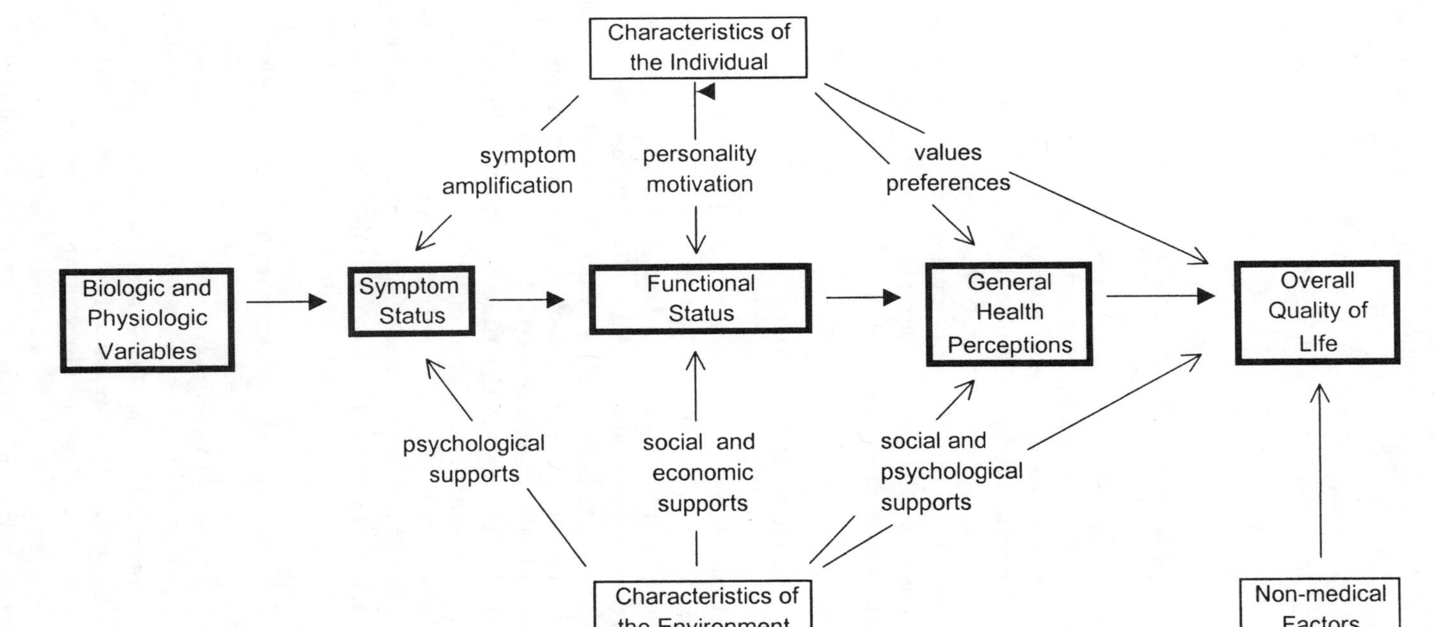

Figure 11.1. Relationships among measures of patient outcome in a health-related quality of life conceptual model. From "Linking Clinical Variables With Health-Related Quality of Life: A Conceptual Model of Patient Outcomes," by I. B. Wilson and P. D. Cleary, 1995, *Journal of the American Medical Association, 273*, pp. 59–65. Copyright 1995 by the American Medical Association. Reprinted with permission.

ity of life (HRQL) will be used to refer to the broad continuum of concepts just described.

What Is the Clinical Meaning of Shift?

In this section I attempt to give a clinical flavor to changes in each of the five types of health outcomes. Note that changes on any scale can be either positive or negative. Examples of biological or physiological change would be the reduction of a blood sugar from 200 to 140 mg/dl, the reduction of a serum cholesterol measurement from 300 to 200 mg/dl, or the increase of a blood pressure from 140/80 to 160/100. Examples of changes in specific symptoms are improvement in the fever and nasal congestion of an upper respiratory syndrome or the abdominal discomfort and diarrhea of a viral gastroenteritis. There are important differences between biological or physiological measurements and symptom reports. The biological or physiological changes just noted are of a magnitude that is unlikely to be perceived. Even if elevated, using population norms as a standard, these conditions are often asymptomatic. An example of change in a specific type of functioning would be recovery from an upper respiratory syndrome or viral gastroenteritis that would enable a child to return to school or an adult to return to work. An example of change in general health perceptions would be the decline in sense of well-being that could occur when a patient is given a new diagnosis of a chronic condition such as diabetes. Finally, an example of change in overall QOL would be declines that could come after a stroke that impairs functioning and general health perceptions (Wilson & Cleary, 1995).

Changes in these different outcome measures, although straightforward when examined in isolation, become complex when two or more dimensions are examined together. Whereas the conceptual model presupposes causal relationships among the five levels of health outcome, the relationships are not necessarily direct or simple (Wilson & Cleary, 1995). For example, as noted, many changes in biological and physiological variables cannot be sensed. Symptoms such as pain may be extremely bothersome at night when someone has no other stimulation and cannot sleep, but minimally bothersome during the day when other stimulations are present. A stroke causing poor ambulation may be a serious problem for a person with diabetes who lives alone and has few financial resources, but it may pose fewer problems for someone who lives with two devoted and healthy daughters and can afford a private nurse. General health perceptions can be low for people newly diagnosed with hypertension, who, with treatment, will have few if any sequelae from the high blood pressure. With time, even the health perceptions of someone with a serious condition, such as a stroke, often improve as the patient learns to accept and live with his or her limitations and develops strategies, both psychological and physical, to cope with disability. Finally, the overall QOL of a deeply religious person who cares more about spiritual than worldly issues may be affected little by physical problems.

What Is the Clinical Meaning of Response Shift?

One way to think about response shift is as relative movement or shift on two or more of the dimensions of health outcome previously described. In theory, two dimensions of health can change in relation to one another in four ways (see Figure 11.2):

1. They can change in parallel.
2. They can change in the same direction, but at different rates or in different amounts.
3. They can change in opposite directions.
4. One can be stable while the other changes.

Consider a 60-year-old lawyer with diabetes who has a stroke that affects his right arm and leg. After completing rehabilitation, he walks

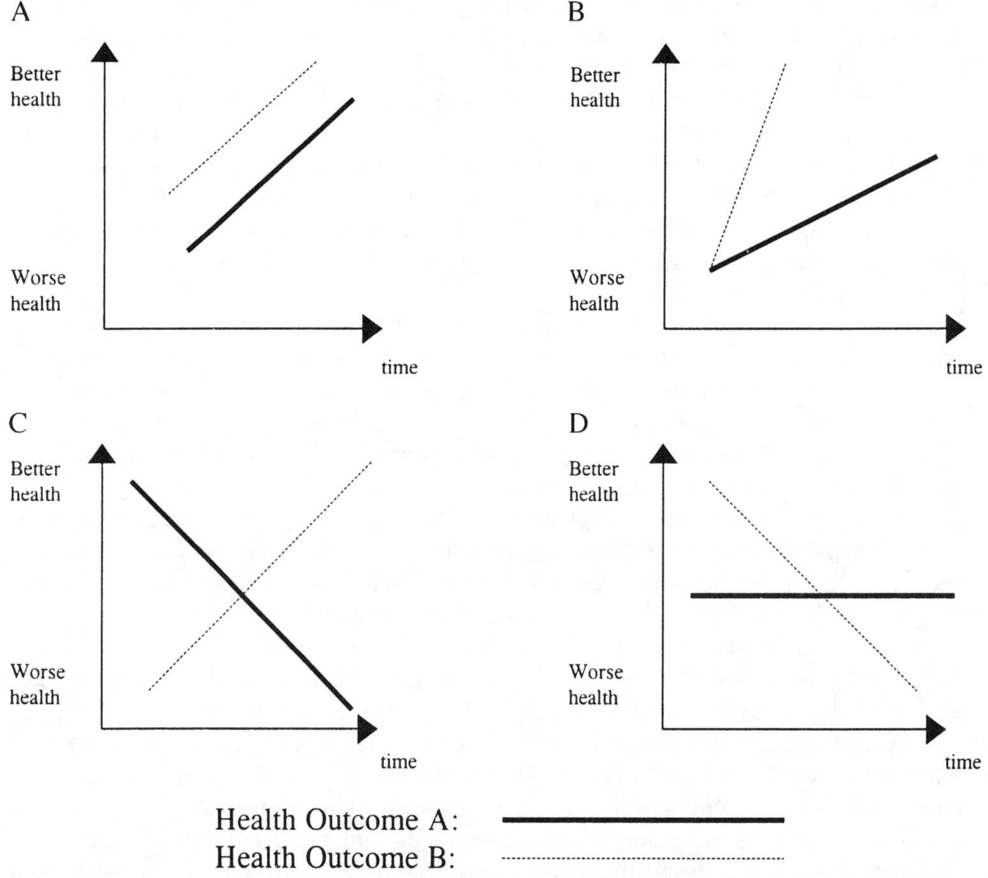

Figure 11.2. The four ways in which two dimensions of health can change in relation to one another: (a) in parallel, (b) in the same direction but at different times, (c) in opposite directions, or (d) one remains stable while the other changes.

very slowly and can barely write, but his cognition is intact. Three months after his stroke, his blood pressure is 170/100 (elevated), and his glycohemoglobin level is 11% (indicating poor blood glucose control over the previous three months). Measures of HRQL reveal that he has a major depression. In addition, his physical functioning, social functioning, general health perceptions, and overall QOL are all quite low.

With help from his family and a private nurse, he is able to return to work. Six months after his stroke he is working half-time practicing law. His blood pressure is still 170/100, and his glycohemoglobin level remains elevated at 11%. Similarly, there has been no improvement in measures of his physical functioning. However, he is no longer depressed, and his social functioning, general health perceptions, and overall QOL have all returned to normal. How did these improvements occur? This man has recovered from the depression that is common in people who have had a stroke, has started socializing with a wide circle of friends, has learned how to do the things he needed to do each day, and has accepted the fact that he had to do things more slowly than previously.

Improvements in this man's general health perceptions would be expected if he were experiencing more strength in his right arm and leg and increasing independence in activities of daily living (ADL). If changes in two or more dimensions parallel each other, there would be no reason to suspect that a response shift has occurred. But here this is not the case; this man's general health perceptions improved even though his physical functioning did not. The simultaneous presence of stability in one dimension with change in another suggests that response shift has occurred. The conceptual point is similar for the improvements observed in depression, social functioning, and overall QOL. In each case, response shift describes changes in some dimensions of HRQL while other dimensions remain static. Note that the specification of relative change is a necessary one. Distinguishing between true change (here called "shift") and scale recalibration, a change in values, or concept redefinition ("response shift") in a particular dimension of HRQL requires reference to another level of health outcome.

Response shifts may be more likely to occur in some levels in the HRQL model than in others. Because biological and physiological variables are in general not determined by self-report, by definition they cannot undergo response shift. Some measures of functioning are concrete and clearly defined—basic ADL, for example—and are unlikely to undergo response shift. For example, one either can or cannot walk up a flight of stairs without assistance. This task is not susceptible to scale recalibration. Similarly, although it is theoretically possible that different flights of stairs are steeper or have better hand rails or better traction, in general a flight of stairs cannot be reconceptualized (concept redefinition). Symptoms, by contrast, can vary in frequency, intensity, bothersomeness, and meaning, and the way that one understands and responds to symptoms can certainly be recalibrated or reconceptualized. General health perceptions are exactly that, "perceptions," and as such are highly susceptible to response shifts. Finally, overall QOL, because it is purposefully subjective, is also highly susceptible to response shifts. Specific, discrete, and objective concepts are less likely to show response shifts than are broad, subjective concepts.

This discussion should make it clear that response shift as it is described here is not a new phenomenon from a clinical perspective. People are constantly in the process of responding to their bodies and the signals they get from their bodies. Medical sociologists have written extensively about the ways in which people perceive bodily sensations, attribute and interpret these physical sensations, and seek care (Mechanic, 1982). When there is a change in health away from the homeostatic state, most people immediately begin the process of response, readjustment, reassessment, and coping. What the concept of response shift does is force us to think about these common clinical phenomena more carefully. Furthermore, response shift potentially gives us new insights into some vexing clinical problems.

The Absence of Response Shift: Somatization and Hypochondriasis

In this section, I argue that physical symptoms are common phenomena in everyday life, that most people have the capacity to adapt to these common physical symptoms, that this adaptation may result in a form of response shift, and that somatization and hypochondriasis are conditions in which this "normal" or adaptive response shifts does not occur.

Population-based studies (Verbrugge & Ascione, 1987) and studies of those presenting for medical care (Garfield et al., 1976; Pilowsky, Smith, & Katsikitis, 1987; Kroenke & Mangelsdorff, 1989) show that physical symptoms are extremely uncommon. The percentage of patients with symptoms that are variously described as functional, insignificant, not serious, or with no identifiable organic origin range from 21–84%. Response shifts may be the result of a normal, adaptive, psychological mechanism for dealing with these common physical symptoms. Over time, with practice, people learn to cope with symptoms of all kinds, often without the help of physicians and health care systems. Sometimes this means that patients perceive a symptom or a set of symptoms but recognize them as transient and representing no serious illness, such as learning to cope with chronic tension headaches or low back pain. Other times this means that general health perceptions and overall QOL gradually improve in the face of fixed physiological problems associated with physical symptoms, such as a patient with osteoarthritis of the knee who learns to cope with both pain and decreased mobility.

The important point is that the symptom perceived by the patient does not disappear. Instead, the patient adapts to its presence. This adaptation may result in a form of response shift. Because functioning, general health perceptions, or overall QOL improve or return to baseline (i.e., "set point"), even though the symptom persists, this process of adaptation is a kind of response shift. Unfortunately, not all people have this ability to produce this type of response shift.

Barsky and Borus (1995) defined *somatization* as "the propensity to experience and report somatic symptoms that have no pathophysiological explanation, to misattribute them to disease, and to seek medical attention for them," (p. 1931). Diagnostic criteria for somatization disorder in the *Diagnostic and Statistical Manual of Mental Disorders*, 4th edition (DSM-IV; American Psychiatric Association, 1994) include the presence of eight individual physical symptoms that have occurred over a period of several years, starting before age 30, and that have caused social, occupational, or functional impairment. Only a fraction of those who exhibit somatization meet criteria for somatization disorder. *Hypochondriasis* is also defined in the *DSM-IV* as a mental disorder characterized by "preoccupation with fears of having, or the idea that one has, a serious disease based on the person's misinterpretation of bodily symptoms," (p. 643) which persists after appropriate medical evaluation. It has been suggested that these phenomena exist along a continuum of tendencies to amplify visceral and somatic symptoms.

For purposes of this discussion, the characteristic feature of these disorders is the rigidity of these patients' conceptualizations of their symptoms, and their resistance to physicians' efforts to reformulate these maladaptive and dysfunctional ideas. As others have reviewed in detail (Barsky & Borus, 1995; Kellner, 1987), somatizing patients are high users of all medical services, including inpatient and outpatient medical, surgical, and laboratory services. They deny the influence of psychosocial factors on their symptoms, disbelieve medical evaluations, resist psychiatric referral, and are refractory to conservative efforts to palliate their symptoms. There are no good therapies for hypochondriasis (Barsky, Geringer, & Wool, 1988; Kellner, 1992), but the most widely tested approaches involve cognitive or educational interventions in which the goal is to alter patients' perceptions about or appraisal of their bodily symptoms. In other words, the goal of treatment is to induce a response shift.

Response Shift and the Placebo Effect

In this section I examine the relationship between response shift and the placebo effect. There is not space to consider placebo effects in detail in this chapter, and interested readers are referred to more detailed recent treatments (Chaput de Saintonge & Herxheimer, 1994; Laporte & Figueras, 1994; Strauss & Cavanaugh, 1996; Thomas, 1994; Turner, Deyo, Loeser, Von Korff, & Fordyce, 1994; White, Tursky, & Schwartz, 1985).

Several authors have offered detailed definitions of placebo phenomena (Brody, 1985; Grunbaum, 1985). These definitions are highly technical, and no clear consensus definition emerges. Brody (1985) has suggested a useful approach by describing three possible explanations for why a patient improves after a given therapy: (a) the "natural history" of the condition; (b) the specific or characteristic effects of treatment; and (c) the "symbolic" effects of treatment, or its effect on the patients' "imagination, beliefs, and/or emotions." The usefulness of this approach to placebo phenomena is that the third explanation identifies a placebo effect rather than simply a placebo. Brody was also careful to place the placebo effect in a larger social and cultural context and identified both physicians and patients as active participants in placebo effects.

Placebo effects have been empirically identified to be present in virtually every healing setting. In a now classic paper, Beecher (1955) reviewed 15 studies of patients with a variety of conditions ranging from seasickness to postoperative pain and found that patients responded to placebos in 21% to 58% of cases, with an average of 35%. Recently Turner et al. (1994) reviewed data demonstrating the size of placebo effects in both medical and surgical treatments, and they emphasized that many studies report effect sizes greater than the 35% average shown by Beecher. Recent reviews of psychiatric treatments showed similar findings (Laporte & Figueras, 1994).

Placebo effects are relevant not just to clinical trials. Consider a patient with a new and bothersome headache whose doctor, after a careful history and physical exam, believes that the patient has a self-limited tension headache. Although it is important to rule out serious intracranial conditions, the physician's main goal in this encounter will be to inform, reassure, encourage, and motivate this patient. To inform and reassure effectively, the physician needs to learn how the patient understands the symptom. For example, it can be valuable to know what attributions and associations the patient has, what the patient's specific worries are, and what the patient's past experiences have been with similar symptoms and treatments. Cultural factors can powerfully affect the type of data the physician needs to collect and how it is interpreted (Helman, 1994; Kleinman, Eisenberg, & Good, 1978). In this case the doctor might ultimately recommend short-term treatment with acetaminophen as an analgesic. However, the primary treatment objectives are to affect the patient's beliefs and emotions about his or her symptoms. Education and reassurance about the etiology and natural history of tension headache, if effective, can alter the level of importance or concern that the patient attributes to the symptom. In other words, they can produce a response shift.

There is conceptual overlap between placebo effects and what others call "interpersonal care." Donabedian (1980) divided the process of care into technical care and interpersonal care. An example of *technical care* is appropriate attention to treatments for which specific pathophysiological mechanisms are known or at least hypothesized. *Interpersonal care* is defined as "the management of the social and psychological interaction between client and practitioner" (Donabedian, 1980, p. 4). Recent useful texts have focused on different aspects of interpersonal care such as physician–patient communication (Roter & Hall, 1992) and the medical interview (Lipkin, Putnam, & Lazare, 1995).

The conceptualization for placebo effects advocated here, in practice, is a definition by exclusion. Therapeutic effects that cannot be attributed to the natural history of the condition or to known pathophysiological mechanisms are attributed to placebo effects. In this light, response shift is one type of placebo effect. Response shift describes a specific psychological mechanism by which patients' self-assessed health can change in the absence of known biological and physiological effects. Conversely, self-assessed health can remain stable in the presence of changes in biological and physiological health. Treatment approaches to somatization and hypochondriasis, which are efforts to produce response shifts in people who cannot do so on their own, are an example of this. The goals of such therapy are not to convince patients that they do not have somatic sensations, but rather to get them to think about them as natural, benign, self-limited, and unassociated with serious underlying illness (Barsky et al., 1988; Kellner, 1992). Such an approach has applications in many therapeutic circumstances.

Response Shift and the Physician–Patient Relationship

A primary commitment of the physician is certainly to apply state-of-the-art science to diagnosing and treating biological or physiological derangements, or disease. Beyond that, physicians should seek to diagnose and treat illness. Illness is variably defined, but it refers broadly to the patient's subjective experience of being sick and encompasses the personal, social, and cultural consequences of sickness (Helman, 1994).

Where does response shift fit into these responsibilities? This is more than a theoretical concern. Every subspecialist has patients for whom science and technology has no treatments or no specific treatments. Many patients, and not only those with terminal conditions, reach the point at which "nothing more can be done," which generally means that all known "conventional" therapies have been tried and were unsuccessful. When the limits of science and technology have been reached, what is left is helping patients understand and cope, to rethink and reframe their experiences, so that they can make the best of their conditions—if not to cure then at least to care. One explicit goal of such care can be the production of response shift. When biological or physiological change is no longer possible, a principal goal of care sometimes becomes the induction of scale recalibration, a change in values, or reconceptualization.

Does this mean that we should attempt to produce response shifts in all of our patients? Of course not. The challenge for the physician in helping patients is to navigate between two extremes. At one extreme is an overly narrow biomedical approach that does not recognize the importance of physician–patient partnerships or the existence of placebo effects. At the other is an approach grounded in misrepresentation or even overt deception. Others addressing this issue have made interesting arguments in defense of paternalism and benevolent deception in the physician–patient relationship (Rawlinson, 1985). Response shifts, no matter how beneficial, never substitute for the timely interruption of damaging biological and physiological processes. Chronic headaches, if produced by an expanding aneurysm, should be treated by a neurosurgeon; persistent low back pain, if produced by vertebral osteomyelitis, should be treated with antibiotic therapy and perhaps surgery as well; and fatigue, if caused by temporal arteritis, should be treated with corticosteroids. A focus on scale recalibration, change in values, and reconceptualization is appropriate only when all such possibilities have been carefully addressed.

Recent research on the use of complementary and alternative medical therapies may provide further insights into response shifts and clinician–patient relationships. Eisenberg et al. (1993) recently showed in a national survey that 34% of Americans used complementary and alternative medical therapies in a given year. The list of conditions for which they sought care included back problems, allergies, arthritis, insomnia, sprains or strains, headache, high blood pressure, digestive problems, anxiety, and depression. The types of complementary and alternative medical therapies used included relaxation techniques, chiropractic, massage, acupuncture, and homeopathy. According to the estimates of Eisenberg et al., patients visit nonconventional therapists more often than they visit all primary care physicians combined and spend out of pocket over $10 billion yearly for these visits, which is comparable to the amount spent out of pocket each year for hospital care. Little scientific research either supports or refutes the benefits of the use of any of these therapies.

So why do patients use complementary and alternative medical therapies? One possible explanation—the explanation naturally favored by practitioners of complementary and alternative medical therapies—is that they are effective. But what does it mean to be effective? Virtually none of these conditions have biological or physiological markers. The success or failure of therapy cannot therefore be assessed by any instrument or machine—only by the patient. Do these therapies achieve true behavioral change, scale recalibration, a change in values, or reconceptualization? On the one hand, practitioners of acupuncture and homeopathy may be dispensing powerful and effective biological and physiological agents that produce true change. On the other hand, they may be dispensing inert placebos that produce "only" scale recalibration, a change in values, or reconceptualization.

More important, what are these practitioners of complementary and alternative medical therapies doing that practitioners of conventional therapies are not? One could speculate that one of the things that they do better is produce response shift. Many complementary and alternative medical therapies use different paradigms of health and disease, and therefore by definition help patients think about their condition in different ways (reconceptualization). When patients have discovered that there is nothing more to be done in the conventional paradigm, complementary and alternative medical therapies may offer another paradigm that both explains a set of bothersome symptoms and offers a whole new set of effective therapies. If such paradigms and therapies are explained and dispensed by a sincere and thoughtful provider, the chances are good that the patient will experience improvement, at least for a while, even if the therapies themselves are biologically inert.

Recommendations for Further Research

In this chapter I have attempted to knit together arguments from several intellectual traditions, and progress in further understanding this topic will depend on interdisciplinary collaboration. For example, scholarly work on placebo effects and physician–patient relationships have little overlap. I have argued that response shift is a construct shared by both of these established research traditions, and it could represent a starting point for collaborative research. Health psychologists, measurement experts, and clinicians all have important expertise to bring to bear in further research on this topic.

More descriptive research can be a starting point for work in this area. Studies that measure concepts from different levels of outcome in the model presented earlier offer us the opportunity to detect and explore disjunctions among different outcome measures. For example, Lubeck and Fries (1993) have presented data showing that the mental health of people with HIV is stable over time, even in the face of worsening physical functioning. However, little is known about why the mental health of some patients with HIV is stable or improves even as their disease progresses, whereas the mental health of others declines. Descriptive studies can lead to the development and testing of specific hypotheses about response shift and its relationship to clinical practice. Because they so often have HRQL problems, patients with chronic conditions are a logical focus for this research.

References

American Psychiatric Association. (1994). *Diagnostic and statistical manual of mental disorders* (4th ed.). Washington, DC: Author.

Armenakis, A. A. (1988). A review of research on the change typology. In R. W. Woodman & W. A. Pasmore (Eds.), *Research in organization change and development* (pp. 163–194). Greenwich, CT: JAI Press.

Barsky, A. J., & Borus, J. F. (1995). Somatization and medicalization in the era of managed care. *Journal of the American Medical Association, 274*(24), 1931–1934.

Barsky, A. J., Geringer, E., & Wool, C. (1988). A cognitive-educational treatment for hypochondriasis. *General Hospital Psychiatry, 10*, 322–327.

Beecher, H. K. (1955). The powerful placebo. *Journal of the American Medical Association, 159*(17), 1602–1606.

Bradley, J. D., Brandt, K. D., Katz, B. P., Kalasinski, L. A., & Ryan, S. I. (1991). Comparison of an antiinflammatory dose of ibuprofen, an analgesic dose of ibuprofen, and acetaminophen in the treatment of patients with osteoarthritis of the knee. *New England Journal of Medicine, 325*(2), 87–91.

Brody, H. (1985). Placebo effect: An examination of Grunbaum's definition. In L. White, B. Tursky, & G. E. Schwartz (Eds.), *Placebo: Theory, research, and mechanism* (pp. 37–58). New York: Guilford Press.

Chaput de Saintonge, D. M., & Herxheimer, A. (1994, October 8). Harnessing placebo effects in health care. *The Lancet, 344*, 995–998.

Donabedian, A. (1980). *The definition of quality and approaches to its assessment*. Ann Arbor, MI: Health Administration Press.

Eisenberg, D. M., Kessler, R. C., Forster, C., Norlock, F. E., Calkins, D. R., & Delbanco, T. L. (1993). Unconventional medicine in the United States: Prevalence, costs, and patterns of use. *New England Journal of Medicine, 328*, 246–252.

Ganz, P. A. (1994). Quality of life and the patient with cancer: Individual and policy implications. *Cancer, 74*(Suppl. 4), 1445–1452.

Garfield, S. R., Collen, M. F., Feldman, R., Soghikian, K., Richart, R. H., & Duncan, J. H. (1976). Evaluation of an ambulatory medical-care delivery system. *New England Journal of Medicine, 294*(8), 426–431.

Greenfield, S., Kaplan, S. H., & Ware, J. E. (1985). Expanding patient involvement in care: Effects on patient outcomes. *Annals of Internal Medicine, 102*, 520–528.

Greenfield, S., Kaplan, S. H., Ware, J. E., Yano, E. M., & Frank, H. J. L. (1988). Patients' participation in medical care: Effects on blood sugar control and quality of life in diabetes. *Journal of General Internal Medicine, 3*, 448–457.

Grunbaum, A. (1985). Explication and implications of the placebo concept. In L. White, B. Tursky, & G. E. Schwartz (Eds.), *Placebo: Theory, research, and mechanism* (pp. 9–36). New York: Guilford Press.

Guyatt, G. H., Feeny, D. H., & Patrick, D. L. (1993). Measuring health-related quality of life. *Annals of Internal Medicine, 118*(8), 622–629.

Helman, C. G. (1994). *Culture, health and illness* (3rd ed.). Oxford, England: Butterworth-Heinemann.

Jacobson, A., Cleary, P., & Baker, L. (1996). The effect of intensive treatment on quality of life outcomes in the diabetes treatment and complications trial. *Diabetes Care, 19*, 195–203.

Kellner, R. (1987). Hypochondriasis and somatization. *Journal of the American Medical Association, 258*(19), 2718–2722.

Kellner, R. (1992). Diagnosis and treatments of hypochondriacal syndromes. *Psychosomatics, 33*(3), 278–289.

Kleinman, A., Eisenberg, L., & Good, B. (1978). Culture, illness, and care: Lessons from anthropologic and cross-cultural research. *Annals of Internal Medicine, 88*, 251–258.

Kroenke, K., & Mangelsdorff, A. D. (1989). Common symptoms in ambulatory care: Incidence, evaluation, therapy, and outcome. *The American Journal of Medicine, 86*, 262–266.

Laporte, J. R., & Figueras, A. (1994). Placebo effects in psychiatry. *The Lancet, 344*, 1206–1209.

Lenderking, W. R., Gelber, R. D., Cotton, D. J., Cole, B. F., & Goldhirsch, A. (1994). Evaluation of the quality of life associated with zidovudine treatment in asymptomatic human immunodeficiency virus infection. *New England Journal of Medicine, 330*(11), 738–744.

Lipkin, M., Jr., Putnam, S. M., & Lazare, A. (Eds.). (1995). *The Medical interview: Clinical care, education, and research*. New York: Springer-Verlag.

Lubeck, D. P., & Fries, J. F. (1993). Health status among persons infected with human immunodeficiency virus: A community-based study. *Medical Care, 31*(3), 269–276.

Mechanic, D. (Ed.). (1982). *Symptoms, illness behavior, and help-seeking*. New York: Prodist.

Norman, P., & Parker, S. (1996). The interpretation of change in verbal reports: Implications for health psychology. *Psychology and Health, 11*, 301–314.

Pilowsky, I., Smith, Q. P., & Katsikitis, M. (1987). Illness behaviour and general practice utilization: A prospective study. *Journal of Psychosomatic Research, 31*(2), 177–183.

Rawlinson, M. C. (1985). Truth-telling and paternalism in the clinic: Philosophical reflections on the use of placebos in medical practice. In L. White, B. Tursky, & G. E. Schwartz (Eds.), *Placebo: Theory, research, and mechanism* (pp. 403–418). New York: Guilford Press.

Roter, D. L., & Hall, J. A. (1992). *Doctors talking with patients. Patients talking with doctors*. Westport, CT: Auburn House.

Strauss, J. L., & Cavanaugh, S. A. (1996). Placebo effects: Issues for clinical practice in psychiatry and medicine. *Psychosomatics, 37*(4), 315–326.

Testa, M. A., Anderson, R. B., Nackley, J. F., & Hollenberg, N. K. (1993). Quality of life and antihypertensive therapy in men: A comparison of captopril with enalapril. *New England Journal of Medicine, 328*(13), 907–913.

Testa, M. A., & Simonson, D. C. (1996). Assessment of quality-of-life outcomes. *New England Journal of Medicine, 334*(13), 835–840.

Thomas, K. B. (1994). The placebo in general practice. *The Lancet, 344*, 1066–1067.

Turner, J. A., Deyo, R. A., Loeser, J. D., Von Korff, M., & Fordyce, W. E. (1994). The importance of placebo effects in pain treatment and research. *Journal of the American Medical Association, 271*(20), 1609–1614.

Verbrugge, L. M., & Ascione, F. J. (1987). Exploring the iceberg: Common symptoms and how people care for them. *Medical Care, 25*(6), 539–569.

White, L., Tursky, B., & Schwartz, G. E. (Eds.). (1985). *Placebo: Theory, research, and mechanisms*. New York: Guilford Press.

Wilson, I. B., & Cleary, P. D. (1995). Linking clinical variables with health-related quality of life: A conceptual model of patient outcomes. *Journal of the American Medical Association, 273*(1), 59–65.

12

Helping Others Helps Oneself: Response Shift Effects in Peer Support

Carolyn E. Schwartz and Meir Sendor

To ease another's heartache is to forget one's own.
—Abraham Lincoln

Although altruism and benevolence are generally considered to be positive traits in an individual, their impact on physical and psychosocial well-being has not been widely investigated. Observational research on other positive traits such as optimism and hardiness has revealed that they can facilitate adjustment to or help protect people from chronic health problems (Peterson, Vaillant, & Seligman, 1988), breast cancer (Carver et al., 1994), acute upper respiratory conditions (Lyons & Chamberlain, 1994), and job-related stress (Howard, Cunningham, & Rechnitzer, 1986). Whereas psychosocial intervention research teaches cognitive and behavioral skills to cope with stressors relevant to the study population, little intervention research has thus far addressed how helping people to focus on and develop altruism and benevolence might influence their own well-being.

In this chapter we describe a secondary analysis of a randomized trial of two psychosocial interventions. Rather than focusing on the outcomes of the supported patients, however (see Schwartz, 1999, for a full report), the emphasis of this chapter will be on the impact of participation on those

---

Adapted from "Helping Others Helps Oneself: An Exploration of the Psychosocial Benefits of Supporting Others," by C. E. Schwartz and M. Sendor, 1999, *Social Science & Medicine, 48*(11), pp. 1563–1575. Copyright 1999 by Elsevier Science. Adapted with permission of Elsevier Science.

This chapter was supported by National Multiple Sclerosis Society Grants FG 880-A-1 and RG 2577-A-2, by Fetzer Institute Grant 563, and Agency for Health Care Policy & Research Grant RO1 HSO8582-02 to Carolyn Schwartz.

We thank Amy Carey for her careful transcription of the focus group discussion, Lawren Daltroy for his help in the planning stages of this study, Elissa Laitin for her help with manuscript preparation and data analysis, and Ajith Silva for his assistance with data analysis. We also thank Carla Chandler, Mirjam Sprangers, and anonymous reviewers for their helpful comments on earlier drafts of this manuscript, and we thank all of the patients who participated in this study.

lay people who were trained to provide nondirective telephone support. This training taught them how to listen actively and to provide a compassionate, unconditionally positive regard to others with the same chronic disease. This work is of an exploratory, post hoc nature intended to facilitate hypothesis generation for future studies. Quantitative and qualitative data are presented to describe a phenomenon that might be replicated in future work.

The existing literature on peer support suggests that helping other people may be beneficial to the helper because it enhances the helper's feeling of self-worth and sense of control, as well as reducing depression (Krause, Herzog, & Baker, 1992; Luks, 1988). Helping others can also be perceived as evidence of self-recovery (Henderson, 1995). Although peer support may be symbiotically beneficial to helper and recipient (Moos, 1986), it can also lead to role strain (Mowbray et al., 1996), emotional contagion (Miller, Stiff, & Ellis, 1988), and burnout (Hare & Pratt, 1988; Weitzenkamp, Gerhart, Charlifue, Whiteneck, & Savic, 1997) if nonprofessionals are not adequately trained (Savishinsky, 1992) or if they lack a positive outlook on caring, have a weak sense of coherence, and report lower levels of hope (Almberg, Grafstrom, & Winblad, 1997; Gilbar, 1998; Sherwin et al., 1992). Maximizing the advantages of peer support may require paying attention to the natural context and process by which relationships develop between people including interpersonal similarity, the consistency of the contact, and developing specific guidelines for the intervention that can reduce the strain and stress of ambiguous roles between helper and recipient (Stein, 1991). In the study described in this chapter, we provided consistent guidelines and supervision and attempted to match helper and recipient on level of education and complementary communication styles.

Response Shift Interpretation of Peer Support

The beneficial effect of helping others may be due to a changing self-evaluation despite no change in objective function or circumstances. This interpretation suggests that a phenomenon known as response shift may be involved. *Response shift* refers to a change in the meaning of one's self-evaluation of a target construct as a result of a change in internal standards of measurement, a change in the respondent's values, or a reconceptualization of the target construct (see chapters 1 and 6). The empirical work presented in this chapter explores the possible role of these three aspects of response shift in the effectiveness of a particular therapeutic strategy. This strategy will be situated within a broader anthropological context drawn from other cultures.

Medical anthropologists have observed that many disparate cultures use a two-step psychological strategy for healing. The experience of illness can be solipsistic, self-absorbed, and focused on internal pain, which limits the patient's psychological resources and can exacerbate the condition (Sendor, 1996). Effective therapy may involve some form of self-transcendence to gain access to an expanded, refreshed sense of self (Sendor, 1996). In many cultures, healing is promoted by encouraging patients to project the focus of their concern away from themselves and toward some other entity (e.g., talisman, amulet, healer, or abstract divine being; Csordas, 1994). This outward motion is followed by a reflexive self-consideration in which they view themselves and their condition from this shifted perspective. In some methods, the projection away from self and reflection back toward self involves patients' conceiving or imagining the illness itself as apart from themselves, then reevaluating themselves in relation to this externalized image to gain a new sense of health (Bilu, 1989; Kleinman, 1980).

A Study of Peer Support in People With Multiple Sclerosis

The outcomes of several psychological interventions will be examined from the perspective of this therapeutic paradigm of projecting outward and reflecting inward. This paradigm will also be situated within the response shift model. The patient population has multiple sclerosis (MS), a chronic autoimmune disease that has a dramatic impact on one's functional abilities and consequently on perceived well-being. This demyelinating disease can affect to varying degrees one's vision, sensation, ambulation, bladder and bowel control, coordination, cognition, and mood (Lechtenberg, 1988; Minden, Orav, & Reich, 1987; Rao, Leo, Bernardin, & Unverzagt, 1991).

We describe a secondary analysis of a randomized trial to explore the impact of being a peer supporter on lay people (n = 5) with MS who provided nondirective telephone support to half of the randomized participants (n = 67). The other half of the randomized participants received a directive group intervention (n = 60). (For a full description of this trial, see Schwartz, 1999.)

Participants had a mean age of 43 years (range 21–61 years). The majority was married, and nearly half were employed. Illness duration ranged from 1 to 37 years, with a mean of 8.2 years. This sample represented a broad range of neurologic disability, with an average level of disability reflecting significant problems with ambulation and involvement of other neurological functional systems. The gender ratio of the randomized participants approximated the general MS population (Martyn, 1991): 73% of the participants were women. In contrast, all of the peer supporters were women.

Procedure. The telephone supporters were five lay people who were trained in active listening and then given a caseload of patients to call once a month for 15 minutes. The peer supporters were identified because they had volunteered to participate in pilot groups in which they had been pretested for coping skills intervention or because they had been recommended as helpful volunteers by the Massachusetts Chapter of the National Multiple Sclerosis Society. All participants were asked to complete questionnaire packets several times over the course of two years. Whereas the randomized participants completed the packets five times in two years, the peer supporters were asked to complete the packets only at baseline, one year, and two years. We compare here only those data collection time points shared by both randomized participants and peer supporters. The last packet for the peer supporters would have been completed when their caseloads were nearing termination.

A focus group was implemented with the peer telephone supporters approximately three years after they had completed their role in the randomized trial. This focus group queried the peer supporters about changes they had noticed over the course of their participation as peer supporters. These qualitative data complemented the quantitative data derived from the questionnaire packet, which addresses quality of life (QOL). The focus group discussion was recorded, transcribed, and content analyzed to identify major themes and experiences reported by the peer supporters.

Peer support training. The peer supporters were trained in active listening and nondirective support and were paid $10 per hour. This therapeutic technique is based on Rogerian client-centered psychotherapy, in which the supporter reflects what the participant says, and does not give advice. The goal is to foster an attitudinal condition such that the individual can find the capacity and the strength to gain insight into and to cope with problems (Korchin, 1976). The specified role was to listen to participants and to help them to explore the feelings they had about whatever they chose to discuss. The peer supporters committed to calling their caseload (5–15 patients, depending on the supporter's availability) monthly for one year, and to being faithful to the study protocol: Telephone calls should not last more than 15 minutes on average, and the supporter must not give advice. Supporters met monthly with the project director to troubleshoot any problems that had arisen in implementing the telephone calls, to reduce the risk of burnout, and to maximize the standardization of the intervention. Caseload assignments were determined by the project director to maximize the compatibility of helpers and recipients. This determination was based on an informal assessment of level of education, personal style, and communication style. Callers and recipients knew only the other's first name and that he or she had MS.

Measures. Three aspects of QOL were examined: role performance, adaptability, and well-being. Role performance was evaluated with the Sickness Impact Profile (Bergner et al., 1976) and the Multidimensional Assessment of Fatigue scale (Belza, Henke, Yelin, Epstein, & Gilliss, 1993). Adaptability was measured by the MS Self-Efficacy function and control subscales (Schwartz, Coulthard-Morris, Zeng, & Retzlaff, 1996), the internal subscale of the Multidimensional Health Locus of Control Scale (Wallston, Wallston, & DeVellis, 1978), and relative profile scores (Vitaliano, Maiuro, Russo, & Becker, 1987) from the Ways of Coping Checklist (Folkman & Lazarus, 1988). Well-being was measured using the depression, anxiety, and social activity subscales from the Arthritis Impact Measurement Scales (Meenan, Gertman, & Mason, 1980), the satisfaction subscale of the Quality of Life Index (Ferrans & Powers, 1992), and the Ryff Happiness Scale (Ryff, 1989). All scores were rescaled for data analysis so that higher scores reflected better functioning.

Statistical analysis. Effect size was computed separately for the two randomized groups and for the peer supporters for each of the QOL outcomes. This formula computes d, the effect size index for *t* tests of means in a standard unit, as follows: $d = |m_A - m_B|/\Phi$, where m_A and m_B are population means expressed in raw units, and Φ is the standard deviation of the population (Cohen, 1988). The means compared were baseline versus one year of follow-up, and baseline versus two years of follow-up. An effect size of 0.2 to 0.4 was deemed small, 0.41 to 0.99 was considered medium, and an effect size of greater than 1.0 was defined to be large. A chi-square test was done to evaluate the association between the total number of small, medium, and large effect sizes by group.

Results

Quantitative. Examination of the outcomes revealed that the peer telephone supporters reported improvement on more outcomes as compared to the patients who received an intervention and that the effect size of these changes tended to be larger than for the latter group ($P^2 = 9.6$, df = 4, $p < .05$). Furthermore, compared to the patients who received an intervention, the peer supporters reported approximately 3.9 times the benefit on psychosocial role performance, 3.5 times the benefit on adaptability, and 7.6 times the benefit on well-being. Specifically, outcomes associated with enhanced confidence, self-awareness, self-esteem, and role functioning showed pronounced improvement among the peer supporters as compared to those participants who received a social support intervention (see Table 12.1). Of note, peer supporters exhibited large improvements in positive outcomes such as self-efficacy, global life satisfaction, personal growth, and purpose in life. They also reported large improvements in negative outcomes such as depression, global fatigue, and physical role limitations. A similar pattern was observed among the peer supporters with regard to other psychosocial outcomes, reflecting small and moderate effect sizes. Although participants who received one of the interventions exhibited change on a number of outcomes, the effect sizes tended to be small or moderate.[1] Finally, peer supporters reported the greatest change in outcomes in the second year of the study (see Figure 12.1).

Qualitative. Participants reported a sense of dramatic change in their lives in a number of areas as a result of going through the experience of being a peer supporter. Content analysis organized the focus group discussion into five major themes that represent the helper's perception of

[1]The statistical method used herein differs in power and efficiency from those used in the primary analysis of the randomized trial, yielding differences in the magnitude and number of statistically significant changes between the two analyses.

Table 12.1. Comparison of Effect Size in a Study of Peer Support Among Patients With Multiple Sclerosis

Quality-of-life outcome	Year 1 effect size (1 year − baseline)			Year 2 effect size (2 year − baseline)		
	Received support	Coping group	Peer supporter	Received support	Coping group	Peer supporter
Role performance						
Social activity	0.81**	0.99**	0.45**	0.58**	0.60**	0.73**
Global fatigue	−0.04	0.15	0.25*	0.08	0.07	−1.04***
Physical role limitations	0.13	0.14	1.60***	0.38*	0.19	0.21*
Psychosocial role limitations	−0.21*	−0.16	−0.56**	−0.25*	−0.33*	−1.14***
Overall role limitations	−0.05	−0.02	0.47**	0.07	−0.07	−0.05
Adaptability						
Self-efficacy function	−0.17	−0.36*	−0.75**	−0.34*	−0.48**	3.18***
Self-efficacy control	0.27*	0.17	−0.97**	0.02	0.12	2.17***
Internal health locus of control	−0.23*	−0.12	−0.20*	−0.07	−0.26*	−0.43**
Problem-focused coping	0.11	0.28*	0.51**	0.17	0.24*	0.35*
Social-support coping	−0.02	0.19	0.15	−0.002	0.002	0.35*
Count-blessings coping	0.44**	0.34*	0.17	0.25*	0.22*	−0.09
Religious coping	−0.06	0.06	0.05	0.10	0.42**	−0.10
Accepting responsibility	−0.17	−0.15	0.72**	−0.005	−0.09	0.25*
Wishful-thinking coping	−0.16	−0.19	−0.80**	−0.15	−0.22*	0.29*
Avoidance coping	−0.03	−0.17	−0.80**	−0.02	−0.11	−0.47**
Blame others	−0.16	−0.31*	−0.57**	−0.24*	−0.45**	−0.87**
Well-being						
Global life satisfaction	0.11	0.18	0.25*	0.18	0.18	9.39***
Autonomy	0.35*	0.36*	3.80***	0.28*	0.35*	4.33***
Mastery	0.11	0.17	1.95***	0.08	0.30*	1.58***
Personal growth	0.22*	0.21*	−0.58**	0.82**	0.71**	2.14***
Social relatedness	0.10	0.27*	0.38*	0.10	0.29*	−0.87**
Purpose in life	0.30*	0.11	0.30*	0.74**	0.52**	1.26***
Self-acceptance	0.16	0.30*	0.71**	0.26*	0.27*	1.08***
Depression	−0.06	−0.05	0.73**	−0.13	−0.05	−0.87**
Anxiety	−0.24*	−0.04	−0.49**	−0.03	−0.16	−0.87**

Note. *Small effect size (0.2–0.4). **Medium effective size (0.41–0.99). ***Large effect size (>1.0).

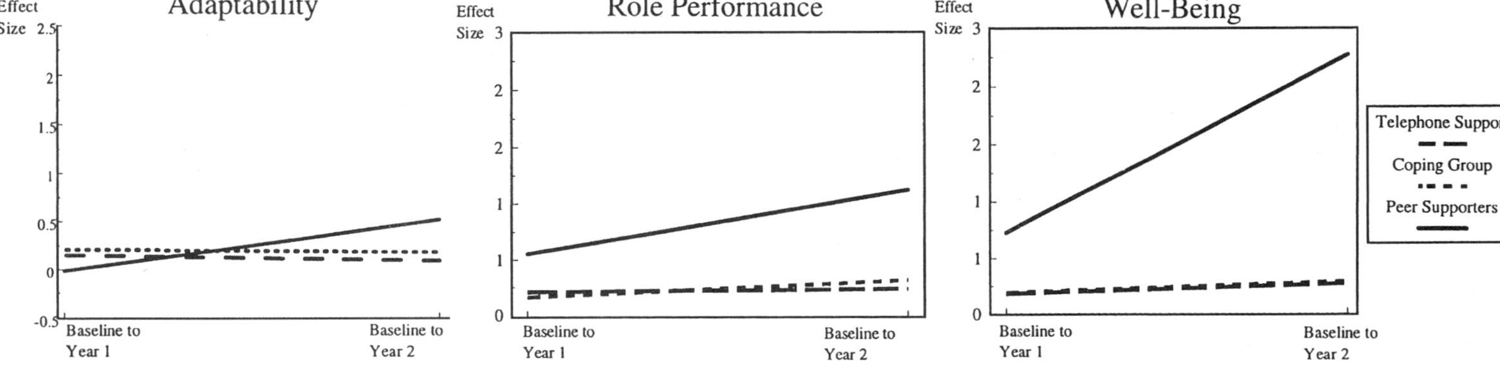

Figure 12.1. Comparison of effect size on adaptability, role performance, and well-being in a study of peer support among patients with multiple sclerosis. The impact of providing support was increasingly beneficial to the helpers over the course of participation.

Table 12.2. Themes Revealed by Content Analysis of Four Groups With Peer-Supporting Patients With Multiple Sclerosis

Sense of having changed	Example
Projection outward	
1. Helper role as self-transcendent	"It's tough to get depressed because you are helping someone."
2. Improved listening skills	"There's a quietness when I'm talking to someone, and I'm really listening to them. I have to make an effort not to try and top them. It's gotten easier. And I can listen, and I become interested in what he's talking about. That's a change. There's a quietness in the soul because of it."
	"There's a comfort in just listening to someone. And instead of formulating something in your own mind, you start concentrating on what you think that person is feeling."
3. Stronger awareness of the existence of a higher power	"I think I've realized that there is a higher power. It's funny, there was a fly on my kitchen window this morning. My husband was going to hit it with the newspaper and I said, 'No, no!' I opened up the window, opened up the screen, and I just kind of . . . because he's flying around, trying to get him down and finally he went out. And my husband said to me, 'What a waste of time. All that time. It took you all that time.' I just looked at him and I said, 'If I take two minutes to help this fly, (laughter) maybe God will take two minutes to help me.'"
Reflection inward	
4. Increased self-acceptance	"I could still feel valuable. Because I could give something. I had something to give."
	"It's not just that you have MS, it's that you have MS and you can help other people with MS."
5. Enhanced self-confidence	"I feel very secure about my future. Not medically, because it can come back any time. . . . I'm not cured. There's no cure for MS, but I really feel like I'm able to handle whatever comes my way."
	"I have a voice that I can speak out. I know what my needs are, and I am able to state what my needs are. . . . It's OK if things don't go my way as long as I know what my way is and that I can verbalize my way."

having changed in the course of the study (see Table 12.2): (a) helper role as self-transcendent, (b) improved listening skills, (c) stronger awareness of the existence of a higher power, (d) increased self-acceptance, and (e) enhanced self-confidence. Whereas the first three themes appear to reflect outer-directedness, the last two seem to be self-referential. First, the role of peer supporter itself shifted their focus away from themselves and toward others. Their affect was attuned not to the potentially negative content of what they heard but to the fact that they were helping someone else. They reported becoming more open and tolerant of others, as well as a sense of inner peace that allowed them to listen to others without judgment or interference. Some also reported an enhanced awareness of the existence of a beneficent higher power. Along with the changes in an external focus were changes in self-reference, reflecting a stronger sense of self-confidence and self-acceptance. For example, supporters mentioned an increased sense of confidence in their ability to manage life's vicissitudes, as well as developing a meaningful context within the constraints of the MS condition.

Discussion

We found that peer supporters reported a greater benefit in QOL outcomes than did those they helped. This effect was particularly pronounced for aspects of well-being and appeared to accelerate during the second year of the study. The increasing benefit of helping others after the first year suggests that supporters adapted to and became more effective in their role, and consequently developed more confidence and gratification from the role. The confluence of the quantitative and qualitative findings suggests that peer supporters were conscious of this improvement. Indeed, they remarked a change in themselves of becoming more outer directed and that this shift changed the way they thought of themselves and enhanced their perception of QOL.

A Theoretical Model of Response Shift Effects in Peer Support

The developing model of response shift (see chapter 1) posits a dynamic feedback loop in which perception of QOL is maintained despite health state changes. This homeostasis is hypothesized to be due to the interaction of antecedent dispositional factors and psychosocial mechanisms that can induce a change in internal standards, values, or concept definition. The central themes revealed in the focus group discussions point to a possible mechanism (see Figure 12.2) within the broader framework proposed by Sprangers and Schwartz.

We propose that response shift is an iterative process of successive approximations that does not happen in one fell swoop. By participating as peer supporters, these individuals were trained to focus on someone else's concerns. Due to the formal, monthly meetings in which peer supporters exchanged stories about people in their caseload, each supporter was exposed to numerous anecdotes and scenarios about other people with MS who were facing challenging situations. This outer-directed role allowed them to disengage from prior patterns of self-reference, and it

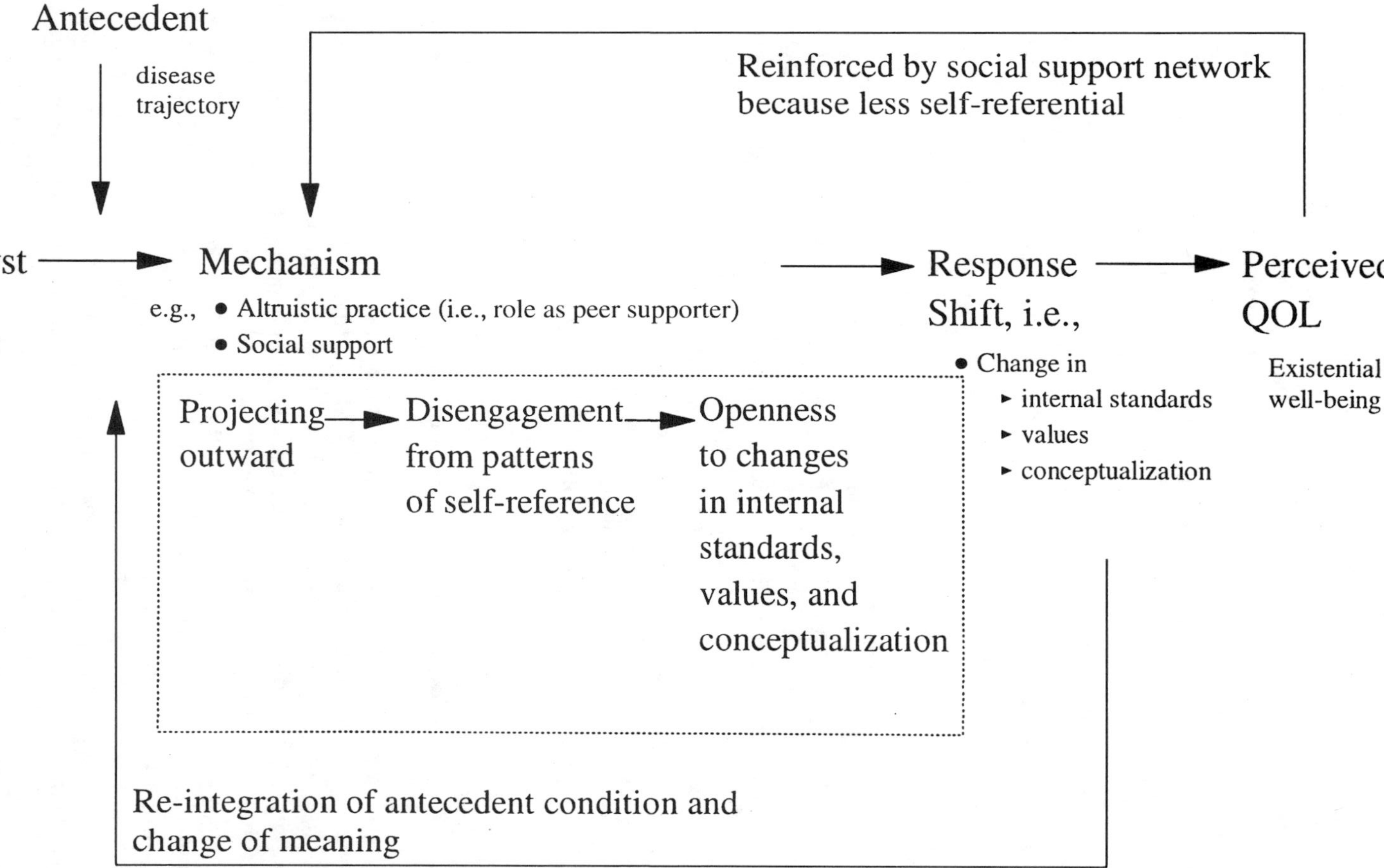

Figure 12.2. A theoretical model of response shift effects in peer support.

thereby facilitated an openness to changing internal standards, values, and concept definition. They could consequently develop a new means of self-reference. Altruistic practice may establish an internal feedback loop that induces response shift. This loop involves projecting outward; disengagement from fixed patterns of self-reference; an openness to changes in internal standards, values, and conceptualization of QOL; and a consequent reintegration of the antecedent condition (i.e., MS) and its personal meaning.

The peer supporters interacted with others who shared the same diagnosis but had different disease trajectories. These interactions may have facilitated a change in internal standards of some aspects of their own MS experience, such as fatigue severity, caregiver burden, or ambulation disability. This change in internal standards may be facilitated by downward comparison (Wills, 1981) or upward affiliative activity (Buunk, Van Yperen, Taylor, & Collins, 1991) caused by the increased exposure to others with the same diagnosis. The enhanced self-esteem reported by the peer supporters in the focus group interview may have protected the peer supporters from negative consequences of upward comparison (Buunk, Collins, Taylor, Van Yperen, & Dakof, 1990). The role of peer supporter may have facilitated changes in values by inducing or encouraging a "communal orientation" (Clark, Ouellette, Powell, & Milberg, 1987). This orientation might have also been reinforced by the expressed warmth and gratitude of the supported patients. Finally, changes in conceptualization might be reflected by the self-transcendence reported by peer supporters (i.e., "It's tough to get depressed because you are helping someone"), suggesting that they had learned new ways of framing their disease experience. Thus even the physical and emotional costs made it easier for them to relate to and help others with the same disease. Involvement as a peer supporter may have thereby induced shifts in all three aspects of the response shift construct.

Although their disease status was not monitored in this study, one can assume that their level of disease activity before they became peer supporters was similar. This assumption is based on research that suggests that the best predictor of rates of exacerbation or disease progression is a patient's own rate during the first five years after diagnosis (Weinshenker, 1994). Thus, improvements in well-being in the context of stable or worsening disease would be consistent with the proposed response shift model (see Figure 12.2).

The mechanism of altruistic practice requires repetition and cumulative reinforcement to influence perceived QOL. This iterative nature is why the mechanism is described as altruistic practice, not one simple act. It is a training process that can have cognitive and precognitive dimensions, because the individual does not necessarily have to be constantly aware of the process for it to occur. Consequently, methods for evaluating response shift might focus more on demonstrating changes in internal standards, values, and conceptualization rather than relying on the self-report of these changes (see chapter 6).

The process of projection outward, disengagement, openness, and reintegration of antecedent conditions is suggestive of the double motion of the therapeutic strategy noted by medical anthropologists, that of projection out and reflection back. This double motion might be particularly suited to induce response shift because of two parameters of the peer support intervention. First, supporters were asked to help others who shared the same medical condition. It may be the case that the efficacy of the projection and reflection is enhanced by the similarity of the object of concern. This similarity may strengthen the identification between helper and recipient and may enhance the reintegration of this antecedent medical condition, thereby changing its personal meaning. It is possible that providing altruistic work to people of vastly different situations would not have the same psychosocial and existential benefit. The second potentially important parameter is the very posture of active listening, which is particularly well-suited to a condition where the threat of increased functional limitations is constant. Engaging in an activity that is feasible to maintain in the face of the possible long-term illness trajectory may further illness accommodation and adaptation. The individual's social support network may also have been strengthened by this developing outer-directedness, as well as by their expanding social role repertoire. The expansion of their listening skills might have been reinforced by others in their social network.

Study Limitations and Future Research

The validity of this analysis is compromised by the possible bias underlying the selection and continuation of the five individuals who accepted the role of peer supporter. Indeed, the peer supporters were selected because of their personal qualities. Additionally, other factors such as the regular group meeting and receiving payment might be interventions themselves and may have influenced study outcomes. Other variables that might influence study outcomes include size of caseload, similarity of background and communication style of provider and recipient, and the fact that all of the supporters were women. Finally, the analysis was post hoc in nature, not planned from the outset of the study. Indeed, the focus group was formed to explore the quantitative findings in greater depth. Consequently the focus group questions presupposed change and perhaps improvement, and they may have led participants to identify changes they might not have mentioned in a different context. All of these factors limit the external and internal validity of the study.

Given the striking nature of our findings, it would be worthwhile to attempt to replicate them in the context of a randomized controlled trial. This trial would assign people to either giving or receiving support based on a specific set of guidelines for matching helper and recipient. It would also measure response shift (see chapter 6), as well as the short- and long-term trajectory in perceived QOL. This randomized trial design could be modified to test the externalization/internalization hypothesis by systematically varying the caseload of those giving support. It would then be possible to investigate a dose–response relationship between size of the caseload and psychosocial outcomes. Competing theoretical models could be tested by operationalizing key constructs that differentiate the various models.

References

Almberg, B., Grafstrom, M., & Winblad, B. (1997). Caring for a demented elderly person—Burden and burnout among caregiving relatives. *Journal of Advanced Nursing, 25,* 109–116.

Belza, B. L., Henke, C. J., Yelin, E. H., Epstein, W. V., & Gilliss, C. L. (1993). Correlates of fatigue in older adults with rheumatoid arthritis. *Nursing Research, 42,* 93–99.

Bergner, M., Bobbitt, R. A., Kressel, S., Pollard, W. E., Gilson, B. S., & Morris, J. R. (1976). The Sickness Impact Profile: Conceptual formulation and development revision of a health status measure. *International Journal of Health Services, 6,* 393–415.

Bilu, Y. (1989). Paradise Regained: "Miraculous Healing" in an Israeli psychiatric clinic. *Culture, Medicine and Psychiatry, 14,* 105–127.

Buunk, B. P., Collins, R. L., Taylor, S. E., Van Yperen, N. W., & Dakof, G. A. (1990). The affective consequences of social comparison: Either direction has its ups and downs. *Journal of Personality and Social Psychology, 59,* 1238–1249.

Buunk, B. P., Van Yperen, N. W., Taylor, S. E., & Collins, R. L. (1991). Social comparison and the drive upward revisited: Affiliation as a response to marital stress. *European Journal of Social Psychology, 21,* 529–549.

Carver, C. S, Pozo-Kaderman, C., Harris, S. D., Noriega, N., Scheier, M. F., Robinson, D. S., Ketcham, A. S., Moffat, F. L., & Clark, K. C. (1994). Optimism versus pessimism predicts the quality of women's adjustment to early stage breast cancer. *Cancer, 73,* 1213–1220.

Clark, M. S., Ouellette, R., Powell, M. C., & Milberg, S. (1987). Recipient's mood, relationship type, and helping. *Journal of Personality and Social Psychology, 53,* 93–103.

Cohen, J. (1988). *Statistical power analysis for the behavioral sciences* (2nd ed.). Hillsdale, NJ: Erlbaum.

Csordas, T. (1994). *The sacred self.* Berkeley: University of California Press.

Ferrans, C. E., & Powers, M. J. (1992). Psychometric assessment of the quality of life index. *Research in Nursing and Health, 15,* 29–38.

Folkman, S., & Lazarus, R. S. (1988). *Manual for the Ways of Coping Questionnaire.* Palo Alto, CA: Consulting Psychologists Press.

Gilbar, O. (1998). Relationship between burnout and sense of coherence in health social workers. *Social Work in Health Care, 26,* 39–49.

Hare, J., & Pratt, C. C. (1988). Burnout: Differences between professional and paraprofessional nursing staff in acute care and long-term care health facilities. *Journal of Applied Gerontology, 7,* 60–72.

Henderson, A. (1995). Abused women and peer-provided social support: The nature and dynamics of reciprocity in a crisis setting. *Issues in Mental Health Nursing, 16,* 117–128.

Howard, J. H., Cunningham, D. A., & Rechnitzer, P. A. (1986). Personality (hardiness) as a moderator of job stress and coronary risk in Type A individuals: A longitudinal study. *Journal of Behavioral Medicine, 9,* 229–244.

Kleinman, A. (1980). *Patients and healers in the context of culture* (p. 243). Berkeley, CA: University of California Press.

Korchin, S. J. (1976). *Modern clinical psychology: Principles of intervention in the clinic and community.* New York: Basic Books.

Krause, N., Herzog, A. R., & Baker, E. (1992). Providing support to others and well-being in later life. *Journal of Gerontology: Psychological Sciences, 47,* P300–P311.

Lechtenberg, R. (1988). *Multiple sclerosis fact book.* Philadelphia: F.A. Davis.

Luks, A. (1988, October). Helper's high. *Psychology Today,* pp. 39–40.

Lyons, A., & Chamberlain, K. (1994). The effects of minor events, optimism, and self-esteem on health. *British Journal of Clinical Psychology, 33,* 559–570.

Martyn, C. (1991). The epidemiology of multiple sclerosis. In W. B. Matthew (Ed.), *McAlpine's multiple sclerosis* (2nd ed., pp. 3–40). New York: Churchill Livingstone.

Meenan, R. F., Gertman, P. M., & Mason, J. M. (1980). Measuring health status in arthritis: The Arthritis Impact Measurement Scales. *Arthritis and Rheumatism, 23,* 146–152.

Minden, S. L., Orav, J., & Reich, P. (1987). Depression in multiple sclerosis. *General Hospital Psychiatry, 9,* 426–434.

Moos, R. H. (1986). Overview and perspective. In R. H. Moos (Ed.), *Coping with life crises: An integrated approach* (p. 25). New York: Plenum Press.

Mowbray, C. T., Moxley, D. P., Thrasher, S., Bybee, D., McCrohan, N., Harris, S., & Clover, G. (1996). Consumers as community support providers: Issues created by role intervention. *Community Mental Health Journal, 32,* 47–67.

Peterson, C., Vaillant, G. E., & Seligman, M. E. P. (1988). Pessimistic explanatory style is a risk factor for physical illness: A thirty-five year longitudinal study. *Journal of Personality and Social Psychology, 55,* 23–27.

Rao, S. M., Leo, G. J., Bernardin, L., & Unverzagt, F. (1991). Cognitive dysfunction in multiple sclerosis: I. Frequency, patterns, and prediction. *Neurology, 41,* 685–691.

Ryff, C. D. (1989). Happiness is everything, or is it? Explorations on the meaning of psychological well-being. *Journal of Personality and Social Psychology, 57,* 1069–1081.

Savishinsky, J. S. (1992). Intimacy, domesticity, and pet therapy with the elderly: Expectation and experience among nursing home volunteers. *Social Science and Medicine, 34,* 1325–1334.

Schwartz, C. E. (1999). Teaching coping skills enhances quality of life more than nondirective behavioral intervention: Results of a randomized trial with multiple sclerosis patients. *Health Psychology, 18,* 211–220.

Schwartz, C. E., Coulthard-Morris, L., Zeng, Q., & Retzlaff, P. (1996). Measuring self-efficacy in people with multiple sclerosis: A validation study. *Archives of Physical Medicine and Rehabilitation, 77,* 394–398.

Sendor, M. (1996, June). *The transforming power of the therapeutic relationship.* Keynote address presented at the "Judaism, Spirituality and Healing Conference" Sponsored by Camp Ramah and the Jewish Healing Center of New England, Palmer, MA.

Sherwin, E. D., Elliott, T. R., Rybarczyk, B. D., Frank, R. G., Hansen, S., & Hoffman, J. (1992). Negotiating the reality of caregiving: Hope, burnout, and nursing. *Journal of Social and Clinical Psychology, 11,* 129–139.

Stein, C. H. (1991). Peer support telephone dyads for elderly women: The wrong intervention or the wrong research? *American Journal of Community Psychology, 19,* 91–98.

Vitaliano, P. P., Maiuro, R. D., Russo, J., & Becker, J. (1987). Raw versus relative scores in the assessment of coping strategies. *Journal of Behavioral Medicine, 19,* 1–18.

Wallston, K. A., Wallston, B. S., & DeVellis, R. F. (1978). Development of the Multidimensional Health Locus of Control (MHLC) Scales. *Health Education Monographs, 6,* 160–170.

Weinshenker, B. G. (1994). Natural history of multiple sclerosis. *Annals of Neurology, 36,* S6–S11.

Weitzenkamp, D. A., Gerhart, K. A., Charlifue, S. W., Whiteneck, G. G., & Savic, G. (1997). Spouses of spinal cord injury survivors: The added impact of caregiving. *Archives of Physical Medicine and Rehabilitation, 78,* 822–827.

Wills, T. A. (1981). Downward comparison principles in social psychology. *Psychological Bulletin, 90,* 245–271.

13

Discrepancies Between Self-Reported and Observed Function: Contributions of Response Shift

Lawren H. Daltroy, Holley M. Eaton, Charlotte B. Phillips, and Matthew H. Liang

Disability is defined as any restriction or lack of ability to perform an activity in the manner or within the range considered normal for a human being (Wood, 1980). A given level of ability, impairment, or function may result in different degrees of disability, depending on the expectations and social roles of the individual. A number of scales with acceptable reliability and validity have been developed to measure disability in performance of instrumental activities of daily living (IADL). They are widely used in research settings, patient care, and general population surveys, including the National Health and Nutrition Examination Survey (Harris, Kovar, Suzman, Kleinman, & Feldman, 1989; McDowell & Newell, 1996). One such scale is the Health Assessment Questionnaire (HAQ; Fries, Spitz, Kraines, & Holman, 1980). The HAQ global Functional Disability Index assesses self-reported limitations in performing 20 activities. Like similar scales, the HAQ is easy to administer, with proven reliability and validity in patient and general populations, but is susceptible to influence in that the respondent's perception of disability is relative to his or her experience and expectations and is subject to response shift in reporting.

Response shift (see chapters 1 and 6) refers to a change in the meaning of one's self-evaluation of a target construct as a result of a change in the respondent's internal standards of measurement (i.e., scale recalibration); a change in the respondent's values (i.e., the importance of component domains constituting the target construct); or a redefinition of the target

Adapted from "Discrepancies Between Self-Reported and Observed Physical Function in the Elderly: The Influence of Response Shift and Other Factors," by L. H. Daltroy, M. G. Larson, H. M. Eaton, C. B. Phillips, and M. H. Liang, 1999, *Social Science and Medicine, 48*(11), pp. 1549–1562. Copyright 1999 by Elsevier Science. Adapted with permission of Elsevier Science.

This chapter was supported in part by National Institutes of Health Grants AR36308 and AG07459 and by the Massachusetts Health Research Institute's Public Health Research Fellowship of the Medical Foundation, Inc. We gratefully acknowledge our collaborator in this research, Martin G. Larson, SD.

construct (i.e., reconceptualization). Social considerations may play an important role in such self-evaluations. For instance, if older people reduce their self-expectations because of gradual loss of function and reduced social expectations, they may be less likely to report difficulty performing a given activity than would a younger person, even at the same objective level of function. This would be characterized as a recalibration response shift (Armenakis, 1988; Breetvelt & van Dam, 1991; Norman & Parker, 1996; Sprangers, 1996), in that the person's internal calibration for difficulty of performance has changed over time. Other influences on reporting may be related to differing internal standards for "difficulty in performing" various activities according to gender, education, social comparison group, or psychosocial function. Susceptibility to such influences and shifts in internal standards may compromise comparisons of disability between populations and tracking of functional ability within people over the life span or disease course.

Many researchers have found considerable discrepancies between self-reported limitations in function in independent ADL and actual physical impairment that is measured as observed function or disease severity (Daltroy et al., 1995; Ford et al., 1988; Kelly-Hayes, Jette, Wolf, D'Agostino, & Odell, 1992; McDowell & Newell, 1996; Ramey, Raynauld, & Fries, 1992; Rubenstein, Schairer, Wieland, & Kane, 1984). A significant portion of the difference between self-reported disability and actual impairment can be explained by demographic, cultural, social, and psychological variables, including gender, familiarity with scale activities, depression, and helplessness (Blalock, DeVellis, DeVellis, & Sauter, 1988; Hidding et al., 1994; Lorish, Abraham, Austin, Bradley, & Alarcon, 1991; McDowell & Newell, 1996). Improved insight into psychological and social factors influencing perception and reporting of disability is important. We may be able to treat disability more effectively if we understand the extent to which self-reported disability reflects true physical limitation rather than the product of psychosocial processes, including response shift, which influence the perception of disability. Study of such differences may also reveal interesting information about how different people evaluate their health.

To explore the influence of social, psychological, and medical factors on self-report of function, we compared a measure of function based on observed performance, the Physical Capacity Evaluation (PCE; Daltroy et al., 1995), with a self-reported measure of difficulty in performing IADL, the Functional Disability Index score of the HAQ (Fries et al., 1980). The goals were to develop and validate the measure of observed physical ability (the PCE) and to test the extent to which variables in addition to observed function would predict self-reported disability. The data also allowed several tests of the response shift phenomenon.

A Study of Self-Reported and Observed Physical Function

Method

Design and participants. The basic methods of this cross-sectional study have been described fully elsewhere (Daltroy et al., 1995, 1999). To summarize, we recruited 289 people, ranging in age from 65 to 97, from low- to moderate-income housing sites for elderly people, rest homes, retirement communities, and private homes. Participants were balanced on age (31%, 65–74; 36%, 75–84; and 33%, 85–97), gender, and geographic region (urban, suburban, or rural). The demographic characteristics of the participants are summarized in Table 13.1. Trained interviewers assessed participants in their homes after obtaining informed consent. Participants provided both self-report of functional limitations (HAQ) and actual performance of physical activities (PCE), with order of assessment determined by random assignment. We collected retest reliability data from a subset one week later. We have previously described development of the PCE (Daltroy et al., 1995) and the influence of psychological, medical, and demographic factors on the discrepancy between self-reported functional limitations and observed physical ability, including response shift (Daltroy et al., 1999). Here we will focus on the response shift data.

Measures. Key study measures included observed function and three aspects of self-reported disability. We assessed physical ability directly with the PCE, which averages performance scores on 13 standardized, normed physical tasks that represent musculoskeletal activities necessary for IADL (flexibility and coordination for dressing, shoulder flexibility, motor facility and ambulation, balance, hand strength, fine motor coordination, and dexterity). Examples of tasks include gripping a dynamometer, putting on a shirt and socks, getting up out of a chair, and walking 32 feet. Scores for each task were rescaled 0 to 100 before averaging, with high scores indicating better functional ability. The scale has high internal and test–retest reliability (alpha = 0.90, r = 0.94).

We assessed self-reported disability with the HAQ (Fries et al., 1980), which also has high internal and test–retest reliability (alpha = 0.90, r = 0.94). The HAQ is based on perceived ability to perform 20 IADL during the past week and is an average of eight subscales (dressing and grooming, arising, eating, walking, hygiene, reaching, gripping, and activities). High scores (on a scale from 0 to 3) indicate the most limited function. Following a modification of the HAQ (Pincus, Summey, Soraci, Wallston, & Hummon, 1983), we used the same format to assess decline over the past six months and satisfaction with function. For each activity in which a participant reported limitations, we asked how much harder it was compared with six months ago and how satisfied the participant was with his or her ability to perform each activity in the past week. We also collected data on age, gender, race, education, occupation, income, marital status, region (urban, suburban, or rural), smoking, exercise (three or more times a week), use of prescription medications (0, 1–2, or 3+), comorbid conditions (sum of 9 conditions, yes or no), hearing and vision problems (yes or no), arthritis (yes or no), pain and stiffness in any joint on the day of the examination (yes or no), depression (using the Medical Outcomes Study Short-Form General Health Survey depression subscale; Stewart, Hays, & Ware, 1988), obesity (body mass index), short-term memory loss (Scherr et al., 1988), illness in the past week (yes or no), a fall in the past month (yes or no), social support (frequency of face-to-face and telephone contact,

Table 13.1. Demographic Characteristics of 289 Participants in a Study of Self-Reported and Observed Physical Function

Measure	% M	(SD, range)
Age in years		80 (7.4, 65–97)
Male gender	46	
White race	95	
Education		
High school or less	34	
Some college	17	
College graduate	49	
Occupation: professional or managerial[1]	51	
Household income more than $20,000/year[1]	48	
Married	40	
Region		
Urban Massachusetts	34	
Suburban Massachusetts	32	
Rural Vermont	34	
Smoke cigarettes	9	
Exercise or walk 3+ times per week	72	
Prescription medications		
0	24	
1–2	41	
3+	35	
Comorbid conditions		
0	13	
1	20	
2+	67	
Hearing problems	41	
Vision problems	25	
Arthritis	46	
Joint pain or stiffness	70	
Depressed (Stewart, Hays, & Ware, 1988) (RAND MOS)[1]	14	
Obese (body–mass index = >27)[1]	18.3	
Memory problems (Scherr et al., 1988) (4+ missed of 12)[1]	39	
Illness in past week	17	
Had a fall in past month	12	
Social support: face-to-face or telephone contact[1]		
Daily	63	
Almost daily	71	
Social support: can get help when needed	86	
Feeling in control of one's life[1]	70	
PCE score		61 (0–86)
HAQ score		.63 (0–2.875)
Dissatisfied with HAQ function[1]		51
HAQ function harder in past six months[1]		42

Note. PCE = Physical Capacity Evaluation. HAQ = Health Assessment Questionnaire.
[1]Modeled as a continuous variable in regression analyses.

ability to get help when needed), and sense of control over life (5-point Likert scale).

Hypotheses. Based on our review of the literature (Ford et al., 1988; Kelly-Hayes et al., 1992; Reynolds et al., 1992; Verbrugge, Lepkowski, & Konkol, 1991; Yelin & Katz, 1990), we hypothesized that each of the variables would be associated with self-reported disability, because of a variety of mechanisms. For example, women tend to report greater self-reported limitations in function than men, controlling for health status or observed function (Davis, Ettinger, Neuhaus, & Mallon, 1991; Harris et al., 1989; Johnson & Wolinsky, 1994; Kelly-Hayes et al., 1992; Reynolds et al., 1992; Thompson & Pegley, 1991). This is perhaps due to differential role demands, perceived importance of the scale tasks, self-confidence, choice of comparison group, or some combination of these (Blalock et al., 1988, 1992; Johnson & Wolinsky, 1994). Dissatisfaction with ability, which has been found to mediate the effect of disability on mental health (Blalock et al., 1988, 1992), was hypothesized to result in increased reports of disability. The various health problems could reduce functional ability directly, but they might also influence participants' perceptions so that they would be more aware of their limitations. This could lead to magnification of disability or could increase the accuracy of reporting, depending on the participants' starting points and psychological mechanisms involved. A recent fall or illness or depression may cause people to underestimate or lose confidence and underuse their physical abilities. The variables marking change in health might be involved in response shift (see hypotheses 2 and 3). The other variables were included in the regression analyses addressing response shift: Because there was empirical or theoretical evidence that they could account for some of the disparity between self-reported and observed function, their presence would reduce bias due to model underspecification.

Although cross-sectional, the data permitted tests of several hypotheses regarding the contribution of response shift phenomena to differences between self-reported and observed function. First, we hypothesized that older participants might be less likely than younger participants to report limitations, especially at low levels of observed function, because of a recalibration response shift. In other words, older people (reinforced by reductions in social roles, social expectations, and ability levels in their age-peer group) would expect less of themselves as they age and would not consider themselves to be limited at the same level as would younger people (with more demanding social roles, social expectations, and fitter peers).

Second, we hypothesized that people with recent loss of function (due to recent illness, a fall, pain or stiffness, or perceived decline in function) would report greater disability at each level of observed function than would those without such losses, because of an inflated perception of limitations. This is based on adaptation level theory (Helson, 1964), which posits that a strong, recent event might have an undue influence on self-perceptions that are based on a moving average of one's experience.

Third, we hypothesized that overreporting of disability because of recent loss of function would be corrected by providing accurate information to participants about their ability. The response shift posited in hypothesis 2 would be counteracted by provision of an external reference point. Thus, we expected that participants tested physically on the PCE first would provide more accurate self-reports than would participants who provided self-report before taking the physical performance test. In other words, participants who could see for themselves what they could do immediately before being asked about similar ADL would be more accurate.

In summary, we expected that gradual loss of function and reduced expectations associated with normal aging would result in a shift toward lower internal standards, with consequent underreporting of disability relative to observed function. A more recent or sudden loss, at odds with a participant's current self-perceptions, would create a shift in the opposite direction, toward overreporting of disability caused by magnification of loss. Finally, provision of an external reference point (a fitness test) would counteract the more recent (and perhaps unstable) response shift caused by the recent loss.

Statistical methods. To test the response shift hypotheses, we first examined bivariate associations between aging and more recent losses and the HAQ disability score (using a probit transformation of HAQ to remove problems introduced by a floor effect). We then constructed a general linear model by stepwise forward and backward regression of the HAQ probit disability score on all variables. Self-reported increase in disability and dissatisfaction with function were then added to create a final model. For hypotheses 1 and 2, we tested the effects of age and more recent losses as main effects. Reasoning that low levels of function might be most counter to expectations among the younger members of our group (representing loss "ahead of time"), we then tested the interaction between age and observed function in predicting HAQ probit. For hypothesis 3, we used the Fisher's Z transformation to compare the simple correlations between HAQ probit and PCE for patients with different order of test administration (HAQ or PCE first). We then examined correlations by type of recent loss (an illness, a fall, pain or stiffness, or perceived decline in function).

Results

Population characteristics. We recruited 289 participants, age 65 to 97; 31% were 65–74 years, 36% 75–84 years, and 33% 85–97 years. The sample profile is reported in Table 13.1.

Measures of functional ability. The mean HAQ score was 0.63 (*SD* = 0.72, range 0–2.875). Thirty-five percent of participants reported no limitations in any activity. We transformed the HAQ score by a probit function to yield a distribution less distorted by the floor effect, and we rescaled them from 0 to 100 (mean = 23, *SD* = 23, range 0–89). The PCE had a

Table 13.2. Association of Measures With Self-Reported Disability (HAQ Probit) Among 289 Study Participants

Measure	Statistic[1]	p
Age	r = .32	.0001
Male gender	t = −4.7	.0001
Education (<high school to postgrad 1–5)	r = −.22	.0002
Region: urban, suburban, rural	F = 6.99	.0011
Smoke cigarettes	t = 1.1	.25
Exercise or walk 3+ times per week	t = −4.0	.0001
Prescription medications: 0, 1–2, 3+	F = 20.6	.0001
Comorbid conditions (0–8)	r = .38	.0001
Hearing problems	t = 2.5	.013
Vision problems	t = 5.0	.0001
Arthritis	t = 6.3	.0001
Joint pain or stiffness	t = 7.6	.0001
Depressed (RAND MOS, 3–17)	r = .34	.0001
Obesity (body–mass index)	r = .06	.35
Memory problems (0–12 missed)	r = .11	.063
Illness in past week	t = 3.0	.0037
Had a fall in past month	t = 2.8	.0073
Social support: contact face-to-face	r = −.16	.0055
Social support: contact on telephone	r = −.04	.49
Social support: can get help when needed	t = −.20	.85
Feeling in control of one's life (1–5)	r = −.25	.0001
HAQ function harder in past 6 months	r = .76	.0001
Dissatisfied with HAQ function	r = .88	.0001
PCE	r = −.72	.0001

Note. HAQ = Health Assessment Questionnaire. PCE = Physical Capacity Evaluation.
[1]r = Pearson product moment correlation coefficient; t = Student's t; F = Fisher's F test.

mean score of 61 (*SD* = 61, range 0–86). Self-reported disability (HAQ probit) and observed function (PCE) were strongly negatively correlated (r = −0.72), indicating that about half of variance was shared. Forty-two percent of participants reported loss of function in the past six months, and 51% reported dissatisfaction with ability in the past week. Both were strongly associated with HAQ (see Table 13.2). To counteract skew in the satisfaction with ability scores, we transformed participants' satisfaction scores by adding one to the total score and taking the natural log. We collapsed sum scores for activities being harder in the past six months (recent decline in function) into not harder (0), moderately harder (1 or 2), and much harder (3 or more).

Hypothesis 1: Response shift is related to gradual aging. As expected, self-reported limitations (HAQ probit) gradually increased and observed function (PCE) decreased with age. However, in a general linear model controlling for observed function (PCE) and gender, the effect of age was not significant. In other words, young elderly and old elderly people made similar self-assessments of functional limitations for a given level of ob-

Table 13.3. Regression of Self-Reported Disability (HAQ Probit) on Subject Measures for 286 Study Participants

Measure	Beta	t	p
Dissatisfied with HAQ function	10.5	13.9	.0001
PCE	−0.43	−9.8	.0001
HAQ function harder in past 6 months	4.0	4.0	.0001
Female gender	3.1	2.9	.004
Joint pain or stiffness	3.2	2.6	.009

Note. HAQ = Health Assessment Questionnaire. PCE = Physical Capacity Evaluation. F = 321.9; df = 5,280; $p < .0001$; $R^2 = 85\%$; $M = 23$; Root $MSE = 8.8$.

served function. Reasoning that low levels of function might be most counter to expectations among the younger members of the group (representing loss ahead of time), we tested the interaction between age and observed function in predicting HAQ probit; this test also was not significant.

Hypothesis 2: Response shift is related to recent losses. Almost all baseline measures were associated at the bivariate level with self-reported disability (see Table 13.2), including several measures of recent loss, such as joint pain and stiffness on the day of testing, recent illness and falls, and decreased function in the past six months. We constructed a general linear model by stepwise forward and backward regression of HAQ probit on all baseline variables. Besides PCE, variables retained in the final model included dissatisfaction with function, increase in self-reported disability over the past six months, gender, and joint pain or stiffness on the day of testing (see Table 13.3). Altogether, these five predictors explained 85% of the variance, an increase of 33% over that explained by observed function alone.

Hypothesis 3: External reference point counteracts response shift. We compared the simple correlations between HAQ probit and PCE for patients with different order of test administration (HAQ or PCE first). Differences by test order were significant. HAQ probit and PCE were correlated more strongly among those who had the PCE first versus HAQ first ($r = -0.81$ vs. $r = -0.63$; Fisher's $Z = 3.24$, $p = .0012$). Further breakdown of these correlations by increases in difficulty over the past six months, falls in the past month, illness in the past week, and pain or stiffness on the day of the examination indicated that the effect in test order was apparent primarily among those who did not report worsening function over the past six months (see Table 13.4).

Among participants whose function had declined, HAQ probit and PCE were correlated similarly whether the HAQ or PCE was first ($r = -0.69$ vs. $r = -0.70$). Among participants whose function had not declined, HAQ probit and PCE were correlated much more strongly for those who had the PCE first versus HAQ first ($r = -0.67$ vs. $r = -0.41$; Fisher's $Z = 2.75$, $p = .006$ for test of whether the difference between the two pairs was

Table 13.4. Correlation Between Self-Reported Disability (HAQ Probit) and Observed Function (PCE) for 289 Study Participants

Measures		Self-report (HAQ) measured first	Observed function (PCE) measured first	Raw difference between correlations
Decline in function in past 6 months	Yes	−.69	−.70	.01*
	No	−.41	−.67	.26*
Fall in past month	Yes	−.60	−.82	.22
	No	−.61	−.80	.19
Illness in past week	Yes	−.68	−.75	.07
	No	−.63	−.67	.18
Pain or joint stiffness on day of exam	Yes	−.64	−.82	.18
	No	−.53	−.74	.21
Total group		−.63	−.81	.18**

Note. HAQ = Health Assessment Questionnaire. PCE = Physical Capacity Evaluation.
*Fisher's Z test for difference between two pairs of correlations, Z = 2.75, p = 0.006.
**Fisher's Z test for difference between two correlations, Z = 3.24, p = 0.0012.

equal). A similar pattern was seen for those reporting illness in the past week versus no illness, but the difference failed to achieve statistical significance.

Discussion and Conclusion

We found that a standardized test of observed function explained half (52%) of self-reported disability in an elderly population, with an additional 33% of variance explained by current joint pain or stiffness, female gender, self-reported increase in disability over the past six months, and level of dissatisfaction with ability in the past week. Our results did not support a recalibration-type response shift due to normal aging (hypothesis 1), at least across this age range (65–97 years). However, our data were consistent with response shift predictions that people recalibrate their self-assessments of functional ability based on recent health problems (hypothesis 2), and that physical performance testing provides salient information for participants who have not experienced recent decline, which can improve agreement between observed function and self-reported ability, perhaps by counteracting a response shift (hypothesis 3).

We hypothesized first that aging might be associated with declining expectations of functional ability, a position supported by attribution research (Rakowski & Hickey, 1992; Rodin, 1986). If this were true, 65-year-olds would report higher levels of disability than would 90-year-olds at each level of function, with the greatest age differences in self-reported disability occurring in the lowest levels of observed function, when loss of function would be most out of line with expectations. However, we found no evidence to support this hypothesis. Controlling for observed function, participants did not differ by age in self-report of disability, nor was there an interaction between age and observed function on self-reports of disability. This differs from the findings of Kelly-Hayes et al. (1992), who reported that participants older than age 75 were more likely than younger people to overreport their disability compared with observed function, results opposite from those predicted by response shift theory.

In our second analysis of response shift, we looked at the effect of perceived decline in function over the past six months. Here we found a very strong effect, consistent with response shift theory. Participants who perceived themselves to have declined (HAQ was harder) reported more disability at each level of observed function than did participants who did not perceive themselves to have declined. A key question, of course, is what is the participant's reference point when asked to report on limitations in ADL—is the reference point age–sex peers or oneself in the distant or recent past? If the comparison is with other people, then social comparison theory may explain the response shift (Breetvelt & van Dam, 1991; Gibbons, 1999). If it is with an earlier version of oneself, which appears to be the case here, then adaptation level theory might apply (Helson, 1964).

In adaptation level theory, people compare each new experience with the midpoint of past cumulative experiences. An event with strong impact or an accumulation of new events pulling in one direction leads the person to reset his or her midpoint to reflect cumulative experience. At the bivariate level, we found that a perceived decline in function over the past six months, a fall within the past month, illness in the past week, and pain or stiffness on the day of the examination were all associated, at high levels of significance, with self-report of greater disability. The first and last of these remained significant even after controlling for other variables. Participants with recent problems such as these might have an inflated perception of their functional limitations that are due to deviation from their internal standard. Their perceptions could be brought into line by self-observation during their participation in the PCE. However, we found no evidence of a consistent directional shift in our analysis of test order effect. We did find, among participants whose function had not declined in the past six months, that correlation between self-reported and observed function was greatly improved when the test of observed function came first, whereas among those whose function had declined, the correlation between self-report and observed function was not affected by test order. This suggests that participants who report recent loss of function might be more aware of their true physical capabilities than are participants without this experience. In other words, recent loss of abilities forces people to assess their own limitations more accurately. Thus, those who have *not* recently lost function may have benefited most from salient information about their abilities that was provided by performing the PCE. This hypothesis is consistent with experimental findings of Sprangers and Hoogstraten (1989), who found that a behavioral pretest canceled an induced response shift, presumably by providing participants with information that enabled them to assess their level of functioning more accurately.

Although our data are limited by the cross-sectional design, results from tests of hypotheses 2 and 3 suggest that performance measures could serve as a universal standard to correct for differential self-report of various subgroups. A practical implication of these findings is that clinicians and researchers should combine self-reports of disability with standardized, observed measures of function, which are less susceptible to perceptual and social influences and response shifts. Further methodological research is needed into ways to combine self-report and performance measures. If putting a physical performance test first improves self-report, as is suggested here, then one could study how much and what type of performance testing results in maximum improvement in self-report accuracy (minimum response shift). A further area of study could be how best to frame physical performance results so as to maximize its informational value to the participant. People concerned about disability after a loss in function might be reassured by a performance test that counteracts a response shift whereby they overestimate their disability. This could possibly lead to reductions in health care expenditures by anxious patients seeking reassurance. These hypotheses would need independent testing.

References

Armenakis, A. A. (1988). A review of research on the change typology. *Research in Organizational Change and Development, 2,* 163–194.

Blalock, S. J., DeVellis, B. M., DeVellis, R. F., & Sauter, S. V. H. (1988). Self-evaluation processes and adjustment to rheumatoid arthritis. *Arthritis & Rheumatism, 31*(10), 1245–1251.

Blalock, S. J., DeVellis, B. M., DeVellis, R. F., Giorgino, K. B., van H. Sauter, K., Jordan, J. M., Keefe, F. J., & Mutran, E. J. (1992). Psychological well-being among people with recently diagnosed rheumatoid arthritis: Do self-perceptions of abilities make a difference? *Arthritis & Rheumatism, 35*(11), 1267–1272.

Breetvelt, I. S., & van Dam, F. S. A. M. (1991). Underreporting by cancer patients: The case of response shift. *Social Science and Medicine, 32*(9), 981–987.

Daltroy, L. H., Larson, M. G., Eaton, H. M., Phillips, C. B., & Liang, M. H. (1999). Discrepancies between self-reported and observed physical function in the elderly: The influence of response shift and other factors. *Social Science and Medicine, 48*(11), 1549–1562.

Daltroy, L. H., Phillips, C. B., Eaton, H. M., Larson, M. G., Partridge, A. J., Logigian, M., & Liang, M. H. (1995). Objectively measuring physical ability in elderly persons: The Physical Capacity Evaluation. *American Journal of Public Health, 85*(4), 558–560.

Davis, M. A., Ettinger, W. H., Neuhaus, J. M., & Mallon, K. P. (1991). Knee osteoarthritis and physical functioning: Evidence from the NHANES I Epidemiologic Followup study. *Journal of Rheumatology, 18,* 591–598.

Ford, A. B., Folmar, S. J., Salmon, R. B., Medalie, J. H., Roy, A. W., & Galazka, S. S. (1988). Health and function in the old and very old. *Journal of the American Geriatric Society, 36,* 187–197.

Fries, J. F., Spitz, P., Kraines, R. G., & Holman, H. R. (1980). Measurement of patient outcome in arthritis. *Arthritis and Rheumatism, 23,* 137–145.

Gibbons, F. X. (1999). Social comparison as a mediator of response shift. *Social Science and Medicine, 48*(11), 1517–1530.

Harris, T., Kovar, M. G., Suzman, R., Kleinman, J. C., & Feldman, J. J. (1989). Longitudinal study of physical ability in the oldest-old. *American Journal of Public Health, 79*(6), 69.

Helson, H. (1964). *Adaptation level theory.* New York: Harper & Row.

Hidding, A., van Santen, J., de Klerk, E., Gielen, X., Boers, M., Geenen, R., Vlaeyen, J., Kester, A., & van den Linden, S. (1994). Comparison between self-report measures and clinical observations of functional disability in ankylosing spondylitis, rheumatoid arthritis, and fibromyalgia. *The Journal of Rheumatology, 21*(5), 818–823.

Johnson, R. J., & Wolinsky, F. D. (1994). Gender, race, and health: The structure of health status among older adults. *The Gerontologist, 34*(1), 24–35.

Kelly-Hayes, M., Jette, A. M., Wolf, P. A., D'Agostino, R. B., & Odell, P. M. (1992). Functional limitations and disability among elders in the Framingham Study. *American Journal of Public Health, 82,* 841–845.

Lorish, C. D., Abraham, N., Austin, J., Bradley, L. A., & Alarcon, G. S. (1991). Disease and psychosocial factors related to physical functioning in rheumatoid arthritis. *The Journal of Rheumatology, 18*(8), 1150–1157.

McDowell, I., & Newell, C. (1996). *Measuring health: A guide to rating scales and questionnaires* (2nd ed., pp. 47–50, 106–115, 335–345). New York: Oxford University Press.

Norman, P., & Parker, S. (1996). The interpretation of change in verbal reports: Implications for health psychology. *Psychology and Health, 11,* 301–314.

Pincus, T., Summey, J. A., Soraci, S. A., Jr., Wallston, K. A., & Hummon, N. P. (1983). Assessment of patient satisfaction in activities of daily living using a modified Stanford Health Assessment Questionnaire. *Arthritis and Rheumatism, 26,* 1346–1353.

Rakowski, W., & Hickey, H. (1992). Mortality and the attribution of health problems to aging among older adults. *American Journal of Public Health, 82*(8), 1139–1141.

Ramey, D. R., Raynauld, J. P., & Fries, J. F. (1992). The Health Assessment Questionnaire 1992: Status and review. *Arthritis Care and Research, 5,* 119–129.

Reynolds, D. L., Chambers, L. W., Badley, E. M., Bennett, K. J., Goldsmith, C. H., Jamieson, E., Torrance, G. W., & Tugwell, P. (1992). Physical disability among Canadians reporting musculoskeletal diseases. *The Journal of Rheumatology, 19,* 1020–1030.

Rodin, J. (1986). Aging and health: Effects of the sense of control. *Science, 233,* 1271–1276.

Rubenstein, L. Z., Schairer, C., Wieland, G. D., & Kane, R. (1984). Systematic biases in functional status assessment of elderly adults: Effects of different data sources. *Journal of Gerontology, 39*(6), 686–691.

Scherr, P. A., Albert, M. S., Funkenstain, H. H., Cook, N. R., Hennekens, C. H., Branch, L. G., White, L. R., Taylor, J. O., & Evans, D. A. (1988). Correlates of cognitive function in an elderly population. *American Journal of Epidemiology, 128*(5), 1084–1101.

Sprangers, M., & Hoogstraten, J. (1989). Pretesting effects in retrospective pretest-posttest designs. *Journal of Applied Psychology, 74*(2), 265–272.

Sprangers, M. A. G. (1996). Response-shift bias: A challenge to the assessment of patients' quality of life in cancer clinical trials. *Cancer Treatment Reviews, 22*(Suppl. A), 55–62.

Stewart, A. L., Hays, R. D., & Ware, J. E. (1988). The MOS short-form general health survey: Reliability and validity in a patient population. *Medical Care, 26*(7), 724–735.

Thompson, P. W., & Pegley, F. S. (1991). A comparison of disability measured by the Stanford Health Assessment Questionnaire Disability Scales (HAQ) in male and female rheumatoid outpatients. *British Journal of Rheumatology, 30,* 298–300.

Verbrugge, L. M., Lepkowski, J. M., & Konkol, L. L. (1991). Levels of disability among U.S. adults with arthritis. *Journal of Gerontology, 46*(2), 571–583.

Wood, P. H. N. (1980). Appreciating the consequences of disease: The international classification of impairments, disabilities, and handicaps. *World Health Organization Chronicle, 34,* 376–380.

Yelin, E. H., & Katz, P. P. (1990). Transitions in health status among community dwelling elderly people with arthritis. *Arthritis and Rheumatism 33*(8), 1205–1215.

14

Associations Between Health Status and Utilities: Indirect Evidence for Response Shift

Leslie A. Lenert, Jonathan R. Treadwell, and Carolyn E. Schwartz

Quantitative evaluations of health states or health values are required in various health services research applications, such as cost-effectiveness studies and medical decision making. For example, in cost-effectiveness studies, valuations of patients' health states are used to adjust survival estimates for appraised quality, resulting in quality-adjusted life years (see also chapter 6). Such analyses require valuations of health states that are independent of those elicited from patients. In other words, the valuations should not be affected by *response shifts*—changes in internal standards, values, or conceptualization of quality of life (QOL) as a function of changes in health (see chapters 1 and 6).

However, there are strong theoretical reasons to suggest that health status and health values should be closely associated with each other and that changes in health should be associated with changes in health values. These reasons have to do with the effects of prospect theory on preferences. Prospect theory is related to response shift theory in that both theoretical models provide mechanisms by which utility values or preferences might change as a function of health state changes. Additionally, both models posit that outcomes are relative to an internal referent. In this chapter we explore the hypothetical effects of prospect theory on preferences and present evidence for strong associations between health status and values.

Prospect Theory and Assessment of Health Values

According to prospect theory, outcomes are evaluated relative to a reference level (Kahneman & Tversky, 1979). In the domain of health quality,

Adapted from "Associations Between Health Status and Utilities: Implications for Policy," by L. A. Lenert, J. R. Treadwell, and C. E. Schwartz, 1999, *Medical Care, 37*, pp. 479–489. Copyright 1999 by Lippincott, Williams & Wilkins. Adapted with permission from Lippincott, Williams & Wilkins.

the most natural choice of a reference level is the person's current level of health. Health states that are better than the reference level are perceived as gains; health states that are worse than the reference level are perceived as losses. Because losses and gains carry different weights in subjective decision making, values for states should differ across different levels of health.

Figure 14.1 illustrates the predictions of prospect theory for effects on values. The x-axis is an interval scale of health state based on measured functional status (not values), anchored at death on one end and perfect health on the other. Consider three intermediate states of health on this scale: being bedridden (C), being wheelchair bound (B), and being able to walk but not having full health (A). Different utility functions could be held by various homogeneous groups of raters for this set of states. Thus, the dashed curve could represent a hypothetical utility function for bedridden patients, and the solid curve could represent the utility function for people who can walk. Prospect theory predicts that utility functions have an S-shaped form, with the inflection point of the curve at the level of health corresponding to a group's current health state. Thus, each group will value transitions between health states differently.

The different shapes of the curves should be associated with differ-

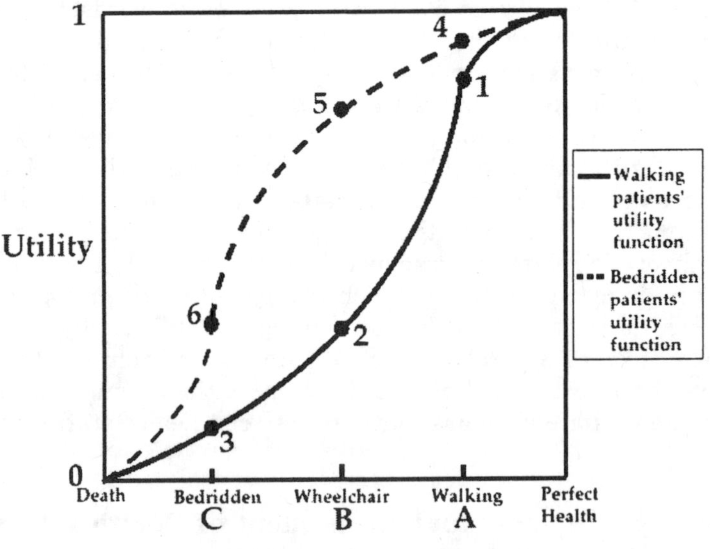

Figure 14.1. Prospect theory predicts that the utility curves for health are S-shaped and that the position of the curve will depend on the reference level of health of the individual. This figure shows two hypothetical utility curves for healthy (solid line) and ill (dashed line) people. There is little difference between healthy people's utility for states B and C (point 2 vs. point 3), which are far below their reference level states. In contrast, for ill people, the difference in utility between will be large (point 5 vs. point 6), because the inflection point in the utility curve occurs at a lower health state.

ences in values for changes in levels of health between groups. For example, consider the change from being bedridden (C) and using a wheelchair (B). Walking patients (whose reference level is point 1) might view this difference as relatively small [(U at point 2)–(U at point 3) is small]. Conversely, bedridden patients may have adapted to this condition and have a reference level at point 4; they would probably view this change as being a significant one.

There is conflicting empirical evidence for effects consistent with prospect theory in measurements of health values. Several researchers have suggested that values for generic health states (such as those seen used in health index models) are remarkably constant across groups (Balaban, Sagi, Goldfarb, & Nettler, 1986; Boyle & Torrance, 1984; Hadorn, Sorensen, & Holte, 1995; Llewellyn-Thomas et al., 1984; Patrick, Sittampalam, Somerville, Carter, & Bergner, 1985). However, other researchers have found important differences in preferences between patients and the general public. These studies have largely focused on utilities for specific conditions (Boyd, Sutherland, Heasman, Tritchler, & Cummings, 1990; Sackett & Torrance, 1978) and show that patients value health states more highly than the general public. Not all studies of utilities for specific health conditions, however, have shown these differences (Clarke, Goldstein, Michelson, Garber, & Lenert, 1997). At least two studies have shown direct associations between health status and utilities. Dolan has noted associations between the level of health of the patient (as measured on the EuroQol health status measure; EuroQol Group, 1990) and visual analog scale ratings for hypothetical states (Dolan, 1997). People in worse health tended to give higher ratings to hypothetical states than did people in better health. Associations have also been reported between preference ratings for current health and hypothetical states (Clarke et al., 1997; Dolan, 1997). Researchers attempting to find direct evidence for effects of prospect theory have found either no evidence (Llewellyn-Thomas, Thiel, & McGreal, 1992) or conflicting evidence (Llewellyn-Thomas, Sutherland, & Thiel, 1993).

Thus, the empirical data on the effects of prospect theory on preference ratings for health states are partially conflicting and incomplete. One weakness of previous studies has been a focus on identification of fixed or main effects of health status on values. However, reality may be more complex. If health status affects the perception of utility differences, observers may see interactions between health status and values without main effects on measurements.

To investigate interactions between preferences and health status, we have applied an approach for assessing response shift—preference mapping (described in chapter 6). The analytic approach we used for the study described in this chapter categorizes the current health of a patient into discrete multidimensional clusters that correspond to the concept of health states. Investigators using this approach first identify the patient's current state based on health status measurements and then test for interactions in value measurements between a patient's current health and his or her values for hypothetical states.

A Study of the Association Between Values and Health

Method

Developing health state descriptions. To study associations between values and health, we created a set of six health states. To create empirically valid descriptions, we studied patterns of health impairment in depressed patients as measured by the Medical Outcomes Study Short-Form General Health Survey (SF-12; Ware, Kosinski, & Keller, 1996). Health states were identified using *K* means cluster analysis of SF-12 mental and physical health scores in a manner described in detail elsewhere (Sugar et al., 1998). We then developed specific descriptions of each of the six states by directly translating the items of the SF-12 into positive and negative statements about the health of people in the state. Each statement reflected the 25–75th percentile of responses to that item by the actual patients. Descriptions of states were made in the first-person singular voice and followed a stylized outline that detailed the QOL of an individual in four domains: (a) physical health, (b) mental health, (c) social activities and personal relations, and (d) work or home responsibilities. The full process of development of the state descriptions is described elsewhere (Lenert, Michelson, Flowers, & Bergen, 1995).

Recruitment. Eligible patients were being seen in primary care practices that were sites of the Partners in Care Patient Outcomes Research Team (PORT) study and who reported symptoms of depression in a screening questionnaire. The study presented here represents a second study in the main PORT study. Patients who (a) had threshold-level symptoms of depression on a screening questionnaire; (b) agreed to enroll in the primary PORT study; and (c) were seen in study clinics in Los Angeles, CA, Columbia, MD, and Annapolis, MD, were given a brochure describing the study. Compensation of $25 was offered for participation.

Data collection. We incorporated the health state descriptions we had developed into a computerized utility elicitation instrument. The computer instrument required patients to (a) provide information about their current health status using the SF-12, (b) rate their current health using computerized versions of visual analog and standard gamble scales, and (c) rate three of six hypothetical health states using visual analog and standard gamble scales. The six health states were divided into three levels: (a) near-normal health; (b) impairments in either mental or physical health, but not both; and (c) impairments in both mental and physical health. Participants rated one state at each level (rather than all six states), which had been selected at random by the computer. This allowed them to rate a full range of health conditions more easily.

In the data analysis, we used patients' reported SF-12 scores to determine the patient's current health state, by identifying the state for which the prototypical SF-12 values were closest to their own SF-12 scores. Visual analog scale ratings were performed on vertical scales implemented with animated computer graphics. The top anchor on each scale was perfect health, and the bottom anchor was death. Standard gamble utility assessments were performed using an approach previously described in Lenert, Cher, Goldstein, Bergen, & Garber, 1998; and Lenert, Michelson, et al., 1995. Patients completed the computerized interview under the supervision of a trained research staff member who assisted them on request.

Data analysis. We performed two sets of statistical comparisons of patients' preference ratings. First, we compared preference ratings for three hypothetical states across three different levels of health status. We analyzed data by the three levels of severity used in our stratified design. To examine the effect of health status on preference ratings, we treated a patient's preference ratings of different states by the same assessment method as was used for independent observations of their preferences. Assumption of independence between ratings for states was reasonable because the protocol measured preferences for states one at a time, and because patients could not see their previous performed preference ratings at the time of providing ratings for the state under evaluation. We used analysis of variance for multiple independent observations to test for differences in state ratings, for a main effect for the health status of the rater, and for interactions between the rater's health status and the level of health of the hypothetical state. Tests of statistical significance were performed based on the Hotelling T statistic (Pillai, 1988).

Second, we calculated the difference between preference ratings for a patient's current health and the most similar hypothetical state. This comparison was performed simultaneously for both visual analog scale and standard gamble ratings using analysis of variance for multiple independent observations. We then determined whether health status appeared to influence the relationship between preference ratings for current health and the most similar hypothetical state.

Results

Of the 153 patients who volunteered to participate, 139 completed the entire computer interview (90%). Most withdrawals from the study were related to failures in Internet communications between the computer program and its remote database. Patient volunteers were middle-aged (mean age 45 years) and predominantly women (67%). About half were currently married (51%), and about a third had been divorced (30%). Patients were predominantly of European ethnic backgrounds (87%). African Americans (8.7%) and Native Americans (4.7%) were the two most common other ethnic groups. The average education level was 14 years of schooling. Most patients were employed on either a part-time or a full-time basis (68%).

Patients reported a wide variety of other medical disorders regarding their current health, including musculoskeletal disease (67%), cardiovascular disease (35%), neurologic disease (31%), pulmonary disease (28%), endocrine disease (24%), mental health other than depression (22%), gastrointestinal disease (19%), and cancer (4%). Most patients (95%) had levels of acute symptoms of depression consistent with a new depressive disorder, and 34% had a history of chronic symptoms consistent with dysthymia.

Mental and physical disorders were reflected in health status measures. The mean SF-12 physical score in this population was 43.8 (SD = 11.0), and the mean mental health score was 37.6 (SD = 11.0). Population norms for both of these scores are 50; the scores observed in this population are typical of patients with depressive illnesses (Ware et al., 1996). The participants were nearly evenly divided among levels of health in the model: 32% in one of the near-normal health states, 28% in one of the moderately impaired states, and 40% in one of the severely impaired states.

As expected, states with lower health status were less preferable than states with better health status. Mean values are shown in Table 14.1. Differences in ratings within participants were highly statistically significant for both visual analog scale [$F(2,137) = 130.7, p < .0001$] and standard gamble ratings [$F(2,137) = 42.6, p < .0001$]. There was no evidence for either fixed effects of health status on visual analog scale ratings or evidence of interactions between health status and particular states. Furthermore, in standard gamble assessments, there was no evidence of a fixed effect of health status on preferences. However, there were statistically significant interactions between the health status of the participant and the state being rated [Hotelling–Lawley Trace $F(4,266) = 2.7, p = .018$] (Pillai, 1988), as is shown in Figure 14.2. This result was due to different preferences for the intermediate states. Specifically, patients in poorer health valued the intermediate state more highly than did patients in better health. This resulted in a larger difference in utility between worst

Table 14.1. Mean Preference Ratings for Levels of Health Measured Using Hypothetical States

	Health state					
	Near normal[2]		Impairment in one dimension[3]		Impairment in both dimensions[3]	
Mean preference rating[1]	*M*	*SD*	*M*	*SD*	*M*	*SD*
Standard gamble utility	0.89	0.19	0.79	0.25	0.71	0.24
Visual analog scale rating	0.84	0.14	0.66	0.19	0.54	0.17

[1]Ratings within individuals for different hypothetical states were statistically different, $p < .0001$, Hotelling–Lawley statistic.

[2]Ratings within individuals performed using different scaling methods for the same health state were statistically different, $p < .02$, paired t test.

[3]Ratings within individuals performed using different scaling methods for the same state were statistically different, $p < .0001$, paired t test.

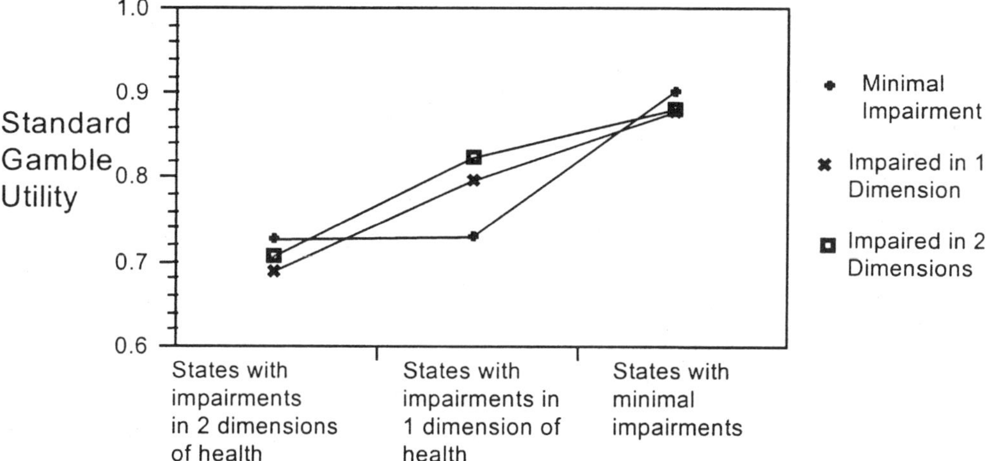

Figure 14.2. Mean standard gamble ratings for different levels of health across participants in different levels of health. Lines connect utilities from different groups with the same levels of actual health (minimal impairments, severely impaired in one dimension of health, or severely impaired in two dimensions). There was no evidence of a fixed effect of level of health on preference ratings. There was, however, a significant interaction between hypothetical levels of health and the actual level of health of the patient ($p = .019$, Hotelling–Lawley statistic). Patients whose own health was in the best category rated the intermediate state lower. Patients whose health was in the worst category rated the intermediate state higher.

health states and the intermediate states in patients with poor actual health than those with good actual health (0.11 vs. 0.001).

Conversely, there were larger differences in utility between hypothetical states with intermediate and good health among patients with good health than among those with health impairments (0.16 vs. 0.055). However, utilities for the best and the worst states were similar across different levels of health status. Seventy-one of 149 patients (48%) rated the state that they were currently experiencing. On average, utilities for current health were similar to those for the closest hypothetical state (95% confidence interval for the standard gamble −0.022 to 0.085; 95% confidence interval for the VAS −0.04 to 0.087).

Conclusion

The study described in this chapter was designed to detect interactions between a patient's current health status and his or her health values. The study demonstrates significant differences in utilities for intermediate states between patients with different levels of health status. However, no effect was found on visual analog scale ratings.

The results of the study appear to support the concept that utility functions for health are S-shaped and differ across levels of health status.

Patients in poor health valued intermediate health states almost as much as near-normal states. Patients in good health valued intermediate states nearly as little as states with poor health. This results in large between-group differences in utilities for changes in good health or poor health to intermediate states.

Interactions between preferences and health status were seen in this study primarily when preferences were assessed using the standard gamble. From the standpoint of evidence for effects of prospect theory, this discrepancy is not surprising, because prospect theory is thought to effect preferences via changes in risk attitude. This might result in minimal changes in visual analog scale scores.

In contrast to standard gamble ratings where there is an interval unit for scaling (1% risk of death), visual analog scale ratings do not have this property. As an individual gains experience with disease, his or her perception of the distance of the state from death might change because of value compression (Dolan, 1997). Compression of the upper end of the analog scale by ill respondents, and of the lower end by well respondents, would tend to offset differences predicted by prospect theory, making detection of effects of health status more difficult with visual analog scale methods.

The results suggest that estimates of effectiveness of an intervention may depend on the health status of the population whose preferences are measured. This finding is consistent with the concepts underlying response shift, and it has important implications for cost-effectiveness analysis. That is, the cost-effectiveness of an intervention will depend on who is rating it. Thus, a small gain will seem more valuable to a person with disabilities than that same gain would seem to a person without disabilities. Consequently, allocation of health resources based on values of the healthy may result in de facto discrimination against those who are ill. These findings have potentially large policy implications (see chapter 15).

This study was conducted in a general medical population with a wide variety of medical problems that were complicated by symptoms of depression. It is possible that depression might alter values in a way that might make the results less generalizable. Previous research on the validity of self-health ratings in mental illnesses suggests that depressed patients may undervalue their QOL in global ratings that use visual analog scale methods (Atkinson, Zibin, & Chang, 1997). Further studies are needed to confirm these findings in populations with other types of health impairments.

Response shift theory suggests that changes in health status should provoke corresponding changes in values, thus relying on a longitudinal framework for study. Because of the cross-sectional design of the study presented here, we are unable to confirm whether values do, in fact, change with changes in health. Rather, this study demonstrates that associations between values and health exist and that changes in values with changes in health are plausible. The time frame for change in health values is unknown, and further work is needed to determine how much lag there is, if any, between changes in health status and changes in values.

References

Atkinson, M., Zibin S., & Chuang, H. (1997). Characterizing quality of life among patients with chronic mental illness: A critical examination of the self-report methodology. *American Journal of Psychiatry, 154*, 99–105.

Balaban, D., Sagi, P., Goldfarb, N., & Nettler, S. (1986). Weights for scoring the quality of well being instrument among rheumatoid arthritics: A comparison to general population weights. *Medical Care, 24*, 973–980.

Boyd, N., Sutherland, H., Heasman, K., Tritchler, D., & Cummings, B. (1990). Whose utilities for decision analysis? *Medical Decision Making, 10*, 58–67.

Boyle, M., & Torrance, G. (1984). Developing multiattribute health indexes. *Medical Care, 22*, 1045–1057.

Clarke, A. E., Goldstein, M. K., Michelson, D., Garber, A. M., & Lenert, L. A. (1997). The effect of assessment method and respondent population on utilities elicited for Gaucher disease. *Quality of Life Research, 6*, 169–184.

Dolan, P. (1997). The effect of experience of illness on health state valuations. *Journal of Clinical Epidemiology, 49*, 551–564.

EuroQol Group. (1990). EuroQol—a new facility for the measurement of health-related quality of life. *Health Policy, 16*(3), 199–208.

Hadorn, D. C., Sorensen, J., & Holte, J. (1995). Large-scale health outcomes evaluation: How should quality of life be measured? Part II—Questionnaire validation in a cohort of patients with advanced cancer. *Journal of Clinical Epidemiology, 48*, 619–629.

Kahneman, D., & Tversky, A. (1979). Prospect theory: An analysis of decision under risk. *Econometrica, 47*, 263–291.

Lenert, L. A., Cher, D. J., Goldstein, M. K., Bergen, M. R., & Garber, A. (1998). The effect of search procedures on utility elicitations. *Medical Decision Making, 18*, 76–83.

Lenert, L. A., Michelson, D., Flowers, C., & Bergen, M. R. (1995). IMPACT: An object-oriented graphical environment for construction of multimedia patient interviewing software. *Proceedings of the Annual Symposium Computer Applications in Medical Care*, 319–333.

Llewellyn-Thomas, H. A., Sutherland, H. J., & Thiel, E. C. (1993). Do patients' evaluations of a future health state change when they actually enter that state? *Medical Care, 31*(11), 1002–1012.

Llewellyn-Thomas, H. A., Sutherland, H. J., Tibshirani, R., Ciampi, A., Till, J. E., & Boyd, N. F. (1984). Describing health states: Methodologic issues in obtaining values for health states. *Medical Care, 22*(6), 543–552.

Llewellyn-Thomas, H. A., Thiel, E. C., & McGreal, M. J. (1992). Cancer patients' evaluations of their current health states: The influences of expectations, comparisons, actual health status, and mood. *Medical Decision Making, 12*(2), 115–122.

Patrick, D., Sittampalam, Y., Somerville, S., Carter, W., & Bergner, B. (1985). A cross-cultural comparison of health status values. *American Journal of Public Health, 75*, 1402–1407.

Pillai, K. (1988). Hotelling's trace. In M. DeGroot, R. Ferber, M. Rankel, E. Seneta, & G. Watson (Eds.), *Encyclopedia of statistics* (Vol. 3, pp. 673–677). New York: John Wiley & Sons.

Sackett, D. L., & Torrance, G.W. (1978). The utility of different health states as perceived by the general public. *Journal of Chronic Disease, 31*, 697–704.

Sugar, C. A., Sturm, R., Lee, T. T., Sherbourne, C. D., Olshen, R. A., Wells, K. B., & Lenert, L. A. (1998). Empirically defined health states for depression from the SF-12. *Health Services Research, 33*(4, Part 1), 911–928.

Ware, J. J., Kosinski, M., & Keller, S. (1996). A 12-item short-form health survey: Construction of scales and preliminary tests of reliability and validity. *Medical Care, 34*(3), 220–233.

15

Discussion: Implications of Response Shift for Clinical Research

Carolyn E. Schwartz and Mirjam A. G. Sprangers

The construct of response shift represents a promising avenue of development for those clinical and social sciences researchers who seek to understand and assess experienced quality of life (QOL) over time. The first section of this book illustrated how considering response shift can illuminate the impact of the illness of oneself or a loved one on one's own well-being. The second section presented methodological frameworks as well as promising avenues of exploration of response shift phenomena. But for many individuals, the true import of response shift is not reflected in the theoretical or methodological intricacies it presents. Rather, it is the sense that the construct has implications for clinical practice and fields related to medical and social sciences. In the last chapter of this first tome on response shift, we would like to mention briefly a few of the implications and future directions for research in the context of observational and intervention research, clinical understanding, and medical decision making. These implications are revealed in many of the chapters, and specifically in the chapters in the third section of the book, in which the authors implemented secondary analysis of existing data to investigate response shift. It is our hope that their example will encourage other investigators to examine their own existing data for evidence and elucidation of response shift phenomena.

When the models and methods of assessing response shift phenomena presented in this book are validated and honed, it would seem likely that we will be better able to understand and assess experienced QOL over time. In chapter 4, for example, Rapkin shows how measuring reprioritization response shift increased the amount of explained variance in QOL outcomes among people with AIDS. In chapter 13, Daltroy et al. illustrate how considering recalibration response shift may improve the correlation between subjective and objective assessments of functional status. Thus, these preliminary investigations support the idea that considering response shift phenomena can improve our understanding and thus our ability to predict experienced QOL over time. Future research might build on this preliminary foundation to examine the contexts in which response shift phenomena are useful or not useful for understanding QOL over time.

A second area of importance is the implication of response shift phenomena on intervention research. Professionals using psychosocial or rehabilitation interventions, for example, may actually *teach* response shift in the context of teaching coping skills for adapting to chronic or terminal illness. For example, they might teach patients more feasible internal standards of role performance given reduced functional abilities (i.e., recalibration response shift). Similarly, they might teach different values and priorities as people's abilities and disabilities change (i.e., reprioritization response shift). Finally, they might seek to teach different ways of thinking about QOL so that patients can maintain a satisfying life quality (i.e., reconceptualization response shift). Whether these shifts are explicitly taught or are inadvertently imparted (see chapter 12), they can lead to striking stability or improvements in perceived QOL despite functional decline. By using a variety of emotion-focused strategies for maintaining well-being in the face of uncontrollable medical illness, these interventions are building on a strong foundation of past research (Vitaliano, DeWolfe, Maiuro, Russo, & Katon, 1990).

A problem arises, however, when outcomes are measured without explicit consideration of response shift phenomena. Results of formal studies might thus reveal only short-term or insignificant effects of interventions. Conversely, preliminary research on the impact of response shift phenomena on treatment evaluations suggests that accurate estimates of treatment gain may be elusive if one does not explicitly measure response shift and that one might actually come to opposite conclusions if one considers response shift (Schwartz, Feinberg, Jilinskaia, & Applegate, 1999). Future researchers might consider response shift in the design phase of the intervention. They might address, for example, how one might best teach response shift and which aspects of response shift are most teachable and effective in buffering perceived QOL from the effects of disease deterioration.

Another type of intervention research that would be influenced by response shift is clinical trials research of medical or surgical interventions. It is likely, for example, that response shift operates differentially in the distinct trial arms and thereby reduces or inflates estimates of treatment gain that are based on the comparability of treatment arms. For example, in a trial of interferon-α for patients with follicular lymphoma, Longo (1998) noted a striking disparity between toxicities reported while patients were on therapy and those reported in retrospect once therapy was stopped. It seems that patients in one arm of the trial had accommodated to the fatigue and low energy level induced by the experimental treatment and had adjusted their performance goals accordingly. Such accommodation made it difficult for the researchers to consider fully the true level of toxicity experienced by the trial participants. Surgical interventions may have similar problems with obfuscation, where patients in distinct treatment arms learn to adapt to the specific drawbacks of the surgery they underwent, leading to no differences in more global assessments of surgical outcome. Such a process might account, for example, for the relatively few differences in reported QOL and body image of women who underwent mastectomy as compared to lumpectomy for breast cancer (Irwig & Bennetts, 1997). By integrating measures of recalibration, reprioritization, and reconceptualization response shifts into trial designs, the response shift effects can be clarified and considered when comparing treatment outcomes.

As our understanding grows of how response shifts are taught or provoked by psychosocial, medical or surgical interventions, the clinical implications of the phenomena will become incrementally more apparent. For example, clinical research might redefine the desired outcome to be the increased disparity between objective and subjective indicators of QOL as patients learn more effective ways of adapting to illness. Clinicians might benefit from considering response shift phenomena as they seek assessment and treatment strategies for clinical phenomena where patients are unable to engage in response shifts (e.g., somatization or hypochondriasis; see chapter 11). For example, they might refer such patients to psychosocial interventions that teach response shift.

Clinicians might also consider the role of response shift in treatment adherence (see chapter 1). For example, patients might evidence low adherence to regimens if they perceive that central values are being challenged by the treatment in question. Clinicians might consequently aim to understand which toxicities or regimen parameters are more tolerable for the individual patients. For example, for young women with lupus, the gastrointestinal side effects of chemotherapy may be preferable to the facial bloating caused by steroids, given a similar impact on relapse. Response shift phenomena may also play a role in the perceived benefits of complementary or alternative therapy interventions, where the scientific mechanism of action is unknown. For example, patients may learn to recalibrate or reconceptualize their experience of the symptom in question, leading to improvements in perceived QOL in the absence of change in clinical indicators of disease.

Response shift phenomena may also influence the experience of pain and other symptoms. For example, patients may learn to recalibrate or reconceptualize their experience of the symptom in question, leading to less impairment in the patient's daily functioning and improvements in perceived QOL. Such response shift phenomena may also play a role in the perceived benefits of complementary or alternative therapy interventions, where the scientific mechanism of action is unknown. Perhaps the success of these interventions is due to the induction of response shift in symptom experience, in the absence of change in clinical indicators of the disease.

Another important implication of response shift phenomena for health-related QOL is related to its relevance to medical decision making. Much cost-effectiveness and medical decision-making work is founded on the use of patient utilities or preferences to determine the most appropriate treatment for them. In chapter 14, Lenert, Treadwell, and Schwartz suggest, however, that patients' life and treatment experiences interact with their preferences. They found that patients in poor health valued intermediate states almost as much as they did near-normal health states, whereas patients in good health valued these same intermediate states nearly as little as they did poor health states. Such disparities can lead to an underestimation of treatment value if healthy population values are used to determine the treatment's cost-effectiveness. Without knowing about the underlying standards that play a role in an individual's assessment of his or her QOL, it makes it difficult to understand how illness affects health.

O'Boyle, McGee, and Browne (chapter 8) suggest that response shift phenomena may lead to reduced validity of advance directives made when a patient is relatively well and death an abstract concept related to the distant future. Similarly, health care proxy judgments may not accurately reflect patients' preferences as patients near the end of life. Other research suggests that patients' retrospective assessment of pretreatment levels of QOL is lower when the treatment is successful than when it is not (Adang, Kootstra, Engel, van Hooff, & Merckelbach, 1998). Furthermore, patients with acute and chronic illness adapt differently (Guadagnoli & Cleary, 1995; O'Boyle, McGee, Hickey, O'Malley, & Joyce, 1992), suggesting that future researchers might seek to elucidate how the course of disease (i.e., improvement vs. deterioration) and its duration (i.e., acute vs. chronic) influences the evolution of patient preferences over time. Such research could be of use for clinicians who seek to guide patients' decisions regarding complex trade-offs between treatments, toxicities, and survival for chronic and terminal illness.

There are many fields of research and clinical practice that are potentially affected by response shift phenomena, and the implications of this impact will become more apparent as our theoretical and methodological frameworks are refined and tested. What is clear, however, is that the phenomena offer exciting directions for researchers and clinicians interested in linking their experience of patients with the clinical indicators they track over the course of their daily practice. It is our hope that this first tome on response shift phenomena points the way to feasible and useful ways of investigating this linkage and of implementing research on response shifts in QOL.

References

Adang, E. M. M., Kootstra, G., Engel, G. L., van Hooff, J. P., & Merckelbach, H. L. G. J. (1998). Do retrospective and prospective quality of life assessments differ for pancreas-kidney transplant recipients? *Transplant International, 11,* 11–15.

Guadagnoli, E., & Cleary, P. D. (1995). How consistent is patient-reported pre-admission health status when collected during and after hospital stay? *Medical Care, 33,* 106–112.

Irwig, L., & Bennetts, A. (1997). Quality of life after breast conservation or mastectomy: A systematic review. *Australian and New Zealand Journal of Surgery, 67,* 750–754.

Longo, D. L. (1998). Interferon toxicity worse in retrospect: Impact on Q-TWiST? [Letter]. *Journal of Clinical Oncology, 16,* 3716.

O'Boyle, C. A., McGee, H., Hickey, A., O'Malley, K., & Joyce, C. R. B. (1992). Individual quality of life in patients undergoing hip replacement. *Lancet, 339,* 1088–1091.

Schwartz, C. E., Feinberg, R. G., Jilinskaia, E., & Applegate, J. C. (1999). An evaluation of a psychosocial intervention for survivors of childhood cancer: Paradoxical effects of response shift over time. *Psycho-Oncology, 8,* 344–354.

Vitaliano, P. P., DeWolfe, D. J., Maiuro, R. D., Russo, J., & Katon, W. (1990). Appraised changeability of a stressor as a modifier of the relationship between coping and depression: A test of the hypothesis of fit. *Journal of Personality and Social Psychology, 59,* 582–592.

Author Index

Numbers in italics refer to listings in the reference sections.

Subject Index

About the Editors

Carolyn E. Schwartz, ScD, earned a bachelor's degree magna cum laude (1982) in psychology from UCLA; a master's degree in clinical psychology (1985) at the University of Connecticut; and a doctor of science degree (1990) from the Harvard School of Public Health, with an emphasis on behavioral sciences, biostatistics, and immunology/cancer biology. She did her postdoctoral training in multiple sclerosis at the Center for Neurologic Diseases of the Brigham and Women's Hospital of Harvard Medical School. She founded and headed the Behavioral Science Research Program (1993–1999) at Frontier Science and Technology Research Foundation (a not-for-profit research foundation) and was a member of the psychiatry faculty at Harvard Medical School (1995–1999). She is currently an associate professor and the associate director of research in Family Medicine and Community Health at the University of Massachusetts Medical School. A specialist in outcomes research and measurement development, her interdisciplinary and methodological research focuses on understanding what patients can do to have an impact on the course of their disease and their well-being. She is on the editorial board of *Psychosomatic Medicine* and the *International Journal of Behavioral Medicine* and is an ad hoc reviewer for numerous journals and granting agencies. She is a Fellow of the Society of Behavioral Medicine and is on the Council of the American Psychosomatic Society. Her publications span the fields of behavioral medicine, health services research, neurology, and oncology.

Mirjam A. G. Sprangers, PhD, earned a bachelor's degree cum laude (1981) in psychology; a master's degree cum laude (1984) in psychological methods; and a doctor of philosophy degree (1989) from the University of Amsterdam, the Netherlands. She has subsequently been a research psychologist at the Netherlands Cancer Institute. She is presently associate professor and vice chair of the Department of Medical Psychology, Academic Medical Center, University of Amsterdam. She coordinates a research line on quality of life and valuation of outcomes that addresses the theoretical and methodological conundrums of health-related quality-of-life and utility research. She is a member of the European Organization for Research and Treatment of Cancer Study Group on Quality of Life and has served as the chair of its Module Development Committee and as a member of its executive committee. She has also served on the board of the European Society for Psychosocial Oncology. She is currently a member of the boards of the International Society for Quality of Life Research, the Dutch Society for Psychosocial Oncology, and the Scientific Council of Social Oncology of the Dutch Cancer Society, and she chairs the Dutch Working Group on Research in Health Status Assessment. She is on the editorial advisory board of the journal *Quality of Life Research* and is an ad hoc reviewer for a number of other journals and granting agencies. Her publications address the methodological, theoretical, and applied aspects of quality-of-life research primarily in oncology and HIV infection.